PHARMACY FINANCE
AND MANAGEMENT
— Your Questions Answered —

Terry Maguire

Pharmacist and Senior Lecturer in Pharmacy Practice

Queen's University of Belfast

Foreword by

Godfrey Horridge

Pharmaceutical Services Negotiating Committee

Radcliffe Medical Press
Oxford and New York

Radcliffe Medical Press Ltd
18 Marcham Road, Abingdon, Oxon, OX14 1AA, UK

Radcliffe Medical Press, Inc.
141 Fifth Avenue, New York, NY 10010, USA

British Library Cataloguing in Publication Data

A catalogue record for this book is available from the British Library.

ISBN 1 85775 153 1

Library of Congress Cataloging-in-Publication Data is available.

Typeset by TechType, Abingdon, Oxon
Printed and bound by Biddles Ltd, Guildford and King's Lynn

Contents

Foreword

Pharmacy Finance and Management – Your Questions Answered is a highly readable book which fulfils a need in the marketplace. It can be read from cover to cover or used as a reference book when questions and problems arise.

It will be extremely useful not only for any pharmacists contemplating purchasing an existing pharmacy business or setting up a new pharmacy, but also for those already running businesses who need a readily available source of advice.

This book will give you a working knowledge of some of the problems encountered but for some of the more complex issues you will still need to consult your accountant or professional adviser.

Godfrey Horridge
Financial Executive
Pharmaceutical Services Negotiating Committee
February 1996

Introduction

I keep six honest serving men
They taught me all I knew
Their names are what and why and when
and how and where and who

Rudyard Kipling, The Elephant Child
Just-so stories (1902)

As pharmacists we are the products of a scientific training that has very little, if any, instruction on finance and business management. Being inquisitive, intelligent individuals we usually learn this aspect of our profession by asking questions either of other colleagues or of professional advisers – mostly our accountants. However, with a lack of structured training in this area and no provision for it in post-graduate training, we can often find ourselves having to make financial and managerial decisions without proper knowledge. In business, ignorance can be expensive.

The roles that pharmacists perform after qualification are very varied but the majority – up to 70% – follow careers in community pharmacy. A pharmacist's career may take a route through management within the multiple pharmacy groups or, after a spell as a manager, he or she may buy a pharmacy and spend his or her career as a proprietor/manager of one or a number of pharmacies.

This book consists of a collection of questions concerning the financial and managerial aspects of community pharmacy practice in the UK. The questions that form the skeleton of the book are those commonly asked by pharmacists. In general the younger pharmacist thinking about, or in the process of, buying his or her first shop has very many financial questions to ask. These questions continue to be asked with great frequency after setting up in business. Equally the newly appointed young pharmacy manager has to struggle with the new world of managing people and resources as well as ensuring that the prescriptions are dispensed. Pharmacists never stop asking questions. As they progress through their careers, financial needs change and even after selling their business and retiring they still need to be concerned about money to maintain their standard of living.

The answers, the flesh of this book, are an attempt to provide sufficient information to empower the questioner to make a decision. When we have the information a decision, either financial or managerial, is so much easier to make.

The book is set out in sections each bringing together the questions that relate to one aspect of the finance or management of community pharmacy. Often the answer to one question may trigger another question and in some sections the reader will find that questions are set out in logical series. No book could hope to anticipate all the financial questions that pharmacists might ask so there may be areas we have missed. I hope these are few.

Whilst every attempt has been made to keep the information in this book up-to-date and as accurate as possible, the world of finance is fickle and can change rapidly. Therefore you must never forget that your accountant or other financial adviser should remain an important source of information.

I wish to acknowledge the many pharmacists who, over the years, have enriched me with their questions, particularly the younger members of the profession that I have had the privilege to teach and who are never short of intelligent questions to ask. It is an arrogant teacher who thinks he knows all the answers. I certainly do not and I am grateful to my many pharmacist colleagues and friends, the many helpful colleagues at the National Pharmaceutical Association, my bank manager and my accountant, whose answers to my questions are contained in the pages of this book.

Terry Maguire
Belfast
February 1996

Basic accounting

QUESTION 1: TYPES OF ACCOUNTS

I am a newly qualified pharmacist and I am attempting to buy a pharmacy. I have been interested in a few businesses and have obtained their accounts. I find them bewildering. Why do they appear so complicated and what do all the different accounts refer to?

ANSWER

They are not so complicated if you know what each item refers to. Financial accounts are required by law and for management and control purposes in a business. They are mainly used to calculate Income Tax or Corporation Tax assessments. Where a business is a limited liability company they are also required to comply with the Companies Act 1985 for; the purposes of auditors, filing returns with Companies House and shareholders who are keen to know how their investments are progressing. Creditors will also have a keen interest in financial accounts.

There are two main types of accounts:

1 Profit and loss accounts – set out the profit or loss for the period. Profit represents the surplus of income over spending and loss represents the surplus of spending over income. Gross profit is the surplus of income after deducting the cost of goods sold. The net profit is the surplus of income after expenses are deducted from the gross profit.

2 Balance sheet – this is a cumulative statement of the financial position of the business. It therefore details how the business is doing over time rather than being restricted to the time period for which the profit and loss accounts refer.

For statutory purposes all self-employed persons and all registered companies must provide a set of accounts annually. More frequent assembly of accounts may provide better management of the business and some businesses will provide accounts quarterly or half-yearly.

QUESTION 2: GOODWILL

In my balance sheet I find that there is a goodwill value of £3000 which refers to the goodwill value I paid for the business 20 years ago. Surely this cannot be correct as the goodwill of the business must be much greater now?

ANSWER

It is normal accounting practice to write off the goodwill value; therefore it would not normally remain in your balance sheet. However, if it is still there your accountant is correct to identify it as the money you paid 20 years ago. He is required to do this due to two basic principles that are used to compile accounts.

The £ standard is the conventional way to express the performance and activities of a business and therefore all businesses are expressed in this money measurement concept. There are, however, a number of disadvantages with this concept since inflation and devaluation are not taken into account which is why your goodwill value is still recorded as £3000.

Assets and liabilities are accounted for on the basis of their historical cost which will not normally equate to current or replacement cost. Current cost being the cost of buying a similar asset of similar age and similar condition and replacement cost being the cost of buying new.

Various attempts have been made over the years to introduce a basis of current cost accounting. However, due to the complexities and the subjective nature of the required estimates implementation has not been achieved.

QUESTION 3: DEPRECIATION – CONSISTENCY CONCEPT

In the past my accountant has always depreciated my fixtures and fittings by the straight line method and my car by a reducing balance method. I have just had a refit and now wish to use the reducing balance method of depreciation as this will give me a greater tax benefit in the first few years. Is this possible?

ANSWER

Normally no. When compiling accounts there is a need to comply with the consistency concept which states that there is consistency of accounting treatment of like items within each accounting period and from one accounting period to the next. It therefore would be incorrect for your accountant to now change the method by which you depreciated your fixture and fittings.

QUESTION 4: ACCOUNTING TERMS

My accountant never seems to have time for me. He is always using jargon that I don't understand and appears irritated if I ask for clarification. Should I just let him get on with it?

ANSWER

I suggest that you change your accountant. You need to appreciate what is going on in your business and your accounts are the best information you can have about this. Like all professions accountancy has developed its own jargon but the meaning of most of these terms is not very difficult to understand. Below I have provided an explanation of the more common accounting terms.

- *Capital* of a business is taken to be the owner's or the shareholders' claim to the assets of the business after other liabilities have been deducted and therefore represents their equity.
- *Revenue* represents sales plus any other income due to the operation of business, i.e. turnover (sales) plus any other income.
- *Capital reserves* represent the permanent capital not available for dividend distribution whereas the *revenue reserves* (*general reserve*) represent an accumulation of past profits available for dividend distribution if required.
- *Expenses* are those costs that result solely from the operation of the business. In other words they are the expenses incurred with the earning of revenue and would include staff wages, lighting and heating.
- *Capital expenditure* refers usually to capital spending from which several accounting periods will derive benefit. Refitting the pharmacy would therefore be regarded as capital expenditure rather than expenses.
- *Assets* are the possessions of the business and can be divided into a number of types.
  - Fixed assets refer to those items required for continuous use in the business and not intended for immediate conversion into cash. Many accounting periods will therefore derive benefit from them. They include land, buildings, fixtures and fittings and motor vehicles.
  - Current assets refer to the cash or other possessions which are intended for ready conversion into cash. Their life is anticipated to be limited and they include cash, stock, debtors, raw materials and work in progress.
  - Intangible assets refer to those items on the books of the business but which have no physical form. These include goodwill and company formation costs.
  - Liquidity indicates how well current obligations can be met with current assets, particularly cash.
  - Solvency is defined as the ability of a firm to meet obligations by using all current assets.
  - Depreciation aims to distribute the cost or other basic value of tangible capital assets, less salvage (if any), over the estimated useful life of the asset in a systematic and rational manner.

QUESTION 5: CALCULATING DEPRECIATION

I do not fully understand what depreciation is and why it appears in both the profit and loss and the balance sheet accounts. Can you explain?

ANSWER

Depreciation is an estimation of how the value of capital items belonging to the business has fallen in the accounting period – usually a year. Since it is regarded as an expense that appears in an accounting period it is classed as an expense to the business and therefore appears in the profit and loss account. The depreciation must also be taken off the value of the capital items; this is therefore noted in the balance sheet.

$$\text{Depreciation} = \text{Deterioration} + \text{Obsolescences}$$

There are two main ways of calculating depreciation – the straight line method and the reducing balance method. To calculate the depreciation of any asset you must establish the cost of the asset, including installation costs, the estimated useful life of the asset, the estimated salvage or resale value and the depreciation method (linear of reducing balance).

1 Straight line method (fixed installment) – this assumes an asset depreciates equally with time. An example is shopfittings which cost £1050 and have a ten year life with a salvage value, when they are sold, of £50. Depreciation may then be calculated:

$$\text{Depreciation} = \frac{1050 - 50}{10} = £100 \text{ per annum}$$

2 Reducing balance method (diminishing balance method) – this assumes that an asset depreciates more rapidly in earlier years. It represents an exponential decay and will go to infinity not allowing an asset to ever be written off. The usual equation used is:

$$\% \text{ rate of depreciation} = 1 - N\sqrt{\frac{\text{salvage value}}{\text{cost of asset}}} \times 100$$

N = number of accounting periods deriving benefit (estimated useful life).

Let us consider again the example of the shopfittings. Using a scientific calculator and the $x^{\frac{1}{y}}$ button it is possible to create the 10th root of the division of 50 over 1050. Here x equals the value and y equals 10. The equation above for reducing balance would read:

$$1 - 0.737 = 0.263 \text{ or a } 26.3\% \text{ reduction per annum.}$$

Year	Depreciation this year	Value of shelving
0	0	1050.00
1	276.15	773.85
2	203.52	570.33
3	149.99	420.34
4	110.54	89.80
5	81.47	218.31
6	60.04	168.27
7	44.25	124.02
8	32.61	91.41
9	24.04	67.33
10	17.71	49.66

QUESTION 6: DUAL ENTRY ACCOUNTING

I have difficulty reading a balance sheet. How does a balance sheet refer to dual entry accounting?

ANSWER

The dual entry system of keeping accounts requires that for every item (a debit entry) there is an equal and opposite item (a credit entry). In its simplest form, let us suppose that you decide to invest £10 000 in a business. The original balance sheet would therefore reflect this.

ORIGINAL BALANCE SHEET			
Owner's equity	£	Fixed assets	£
You	10 000		–
Current liabilities		Current assets	
	–		10 000
	10 000		10 000

Figure 1 Original balance sheet showing dual entry accounting.

This balance sheet accounts for the origin of the capital and shows that, whereas the assets of the business are £10 000, it is offset by an equity claim from the owner.

For the purpose of a cash-based business such as a community pharmacy a summarized version of the dual entry system is used.

Buying a pharmacy

QUESTION 7: BUYING A PHARMACY

I have got the accounts of a pharmacy that I am keen to buy. How can I come to a realistic offer price so that I might be considered a serious bidder but be sure that I am not offering too much?

ANSWER

Unfortunately this is not an exact science with a predetermined formula. There will be three main elements to the purchase:

1 goodwill
2 fixtures and fittings
3 stock.

The recommendation for goodwill is a yardstick around which the parties can negotiate. However, as with most major purchases in your life it will be a matter of what the purchaser will pay and what the vendor will accept. To help value a business, accountants will often weight the relative value of past profits so that this year's profit would be weighted relatively higher than the equivalent profit of three years ago.

Traditionally goodwill was calculated financially to represent three to five years of real net profit. The assumption was that if you were starting a business from scratch then it would take this time to reach the real net profit that this business has obtained.

For community pharmacies this has changed since there is now a limitation on where a new pharmacy with a dispensing contract can be opened. This puts a premium on pharmacies and often goodwill values can be as high as 80 pence per £ of turnover, i.e. if the business turned £200 000 of business in the year you could be paying £160 000 for goodwill.

These are the exceptions however and most pharmacies will change hands with a goodwill value of 35 to 45 pence per £ of turnover.

Goodwill should take into account the cost of rent (a high rent will reduce the goodwill value) and the number of prescriptions. Since there is a threshold above which a professional allowance is paid then pharmacies below this figure will have low goodwill values. Goodwill values are heavily influenced by location, i.e. prime sites will attract the highest goodwill values.

The percentage gross profit should ideally be as high as possible but can range from 15% to 35%. The average pharmacy will return a gross profit of between 20% and 25%. Since the margin on NHS dispensing is now about 16% profit on return, a low gross profit may reflect high NHS dispensing with little front counter business. Profit from front counter business in the average pharmacy can be about 26%. The ideal mix is now about 50% counter and 50% NHS but this is rarely achieved by independent contractors who usually have a mix of 25% counter and 75% NHS. Where the counter percentage is too high this could mean that competition from a non-pharmacy business is imminent and this would necessitate cutting margins to compete.

QUESTION 8: BUSINESS PLANNING

I have been asked by my bank manager to submit a business plan to support a request for a loan. What elements should I include in my plan?

ANSWER

A business plan is a written statement of a proposed strategy for a business enterprise. It might be a proposal to buy, set up or expand a business. A business plan includes the personal philosophy of the owner, a financial description of the business, methods of financing, growth projections and clearly defined management policies in key areas.

A personal business plan is never a static thing and will constantly evolve and change as you develop. It will force you to consider competitive conditions, promotional strategies, best and worst case scenarios and contingency planning.

The components of a business plan are: personal financial goals and objectives; your management experience; personal attributes (positive and negative); a detailed description of the business; and a financial description of the business.

The most important section of the plan concerns the financial description. In this you must demonstrate how the business will generate profit to ensure its on-going financial viability. If you are getting a loan you must demonstrate how you can afford to repay the loan, pay the expenses of the business and also have something left over to live on while leaving working capital to run the business in the first few years. The major source of business failures, including pharmacy business failures, is undercapitalizing. Borrowing just enough to buy the business may be your first mistake.

In this section of your business plan you should include a balance sheet statement, an income statement and a cash-flow projection. This will be based on the current trends you have noted in the area and on the performance in the last three years of the business.

You will be expected to present a profit and loss account and balance sheet for the business for at least three years and a statement of payment from the Health Authority (Health Boards in Scotland and CSA in Northern Ireland).

In your projections the first year should be broken down into months and thereafter annually for up to ten years depending on what your preferred repayment period is. A number of spreadsheet computer programs are available for making projections and your accountant or your wholesaler may provide you with this service.

Income projection is a moving financial picture of your pharmacy. It shows the monthly flow of income, expenses, profit and loss. It shows operating expenses such as rent, labour, supplies and advertising plus cost of goods sold, subtracted from a reasonable estimate of gross sales for a given period.

Cash-flow projection forecasts the actual cash surplus or deficit for each period. While the income statement shows recorded cash and credit sales and all expenses, a cash-flow statement shows items such as payments on loans and withdrawals by the owner.

The income statement will contain accrued income and expenses for the period while the cash-flow statement outlines the actual cash received. Items such as depreciation will appear in the income statement but since it is a notional cost not involving outflows of money it will not appear in the cash-flow statement. At this point a thorough appreciation of the concept of accruals accounting is beneficial.

A projected cash deficit (negative cash-flow) in any period may signal a need to arrange for additional funds to cover the deficit, discuss with suppliers the possibility of extending credit terms or decrease an optional expenditure, e.g. do not withdraw a wage.

During the first year of business, in a time of expansion or any time finances require close scrutiny, these financial projections should be recorded monthly. Later, quarterly income and cash-flow statements should be sufficient to keep the owner/manager knowledgeable of the pharmacy's performance.

It is foolish when presenting projected figures to do so with enthusiasm and be overly optimistic. A bank manager or other financial adviser will soon spot this and it will hinder your ability to secure a loan. It is best to be conservative and prepare for a worst case scenario.

QUESTION 9: INTEREST PAYMENT

I am preparing a business plan but I am not sure how much I will be repaying on my loan since, at this stage, I have no idea what my loan will be. This will depend on how much I eventually pay for the business. Is there a rough guide to calculating interest payments?

ANSWER

Tables are available that show the monthly repayment for a range of interest rates. They are normally only available within the bank. You will be repaying both capital and interest on a monthly basis and as your capital falls so does your interest rate. On a £200 000 loan over ten years at an interest rate of about 9% you will be repaying £2500 per month or £30 000 per year.

QUESTION 10: BORROWING MONEY

I am buying a pharmacy and will need a loan for most of the money. Who will lend me money and what are their relative merits?

ANSWER

Most pharmacy businesses do not fail and therefore they would appear to be a good option for most investment groups. However, recent market problems which have shown that even the strongest business can fail have prompted caution in all sectors of the money market. Over the past decade the fluctuation of interest rates and goodwill values have made the financing of independent community pharmacies more difficult and unpredictable.

It will be very rare to have a financial venture funded 100% by someone else. You will be required to take some risks and this will depend on what you have at your disposal. Most banks will require the full loan to be secured. You may own a property which they can take a charge over, you might have an insurance policy in case of death or you might be required to put up a percentage of the cash. This could be anywhere from 10% to 40% of the loan depending on your circumstances. In particular, a lending agency is less comfortable when paying for intangible assets such as goodwill than they are when paying for a tangible asset like stock or the building.

The bank is the most obvious source of finance for an individual pharmacist and their attitudes towards funding pharmacy ventures has improved over recent years. If you have been banking with a bank for some years, the manager will know your pedigree and this will be a major benefit when an application is decided. They will require a detailed description of the business and how you intend to repay the loan. Additionally, they will require security but this may be negotiable.

You will need to negotiate the interest rate and this can be set between 1.5% and 3% above base rate – the base rate is set by the Government and is traditionally taken as the cost to the bank of making the money available. In a large loan of, say, £200 000 a difference of 0.5% in the interest rate is considerable – so you must negotiate. Additionally, there will be a settlement fee – this is usually 1% of the loan value but your bank manager has a certain latitude here and again you should negotiate firmly.

Obviously, the banks are in the business of lending money and you can negotiate. The more certain an enterprise is the more negotiating space you have and most pharmacies fall into this category. The favoured method of repayment is by capital plus interest calculated over a defined period. Of course the interest rate is likely to alter with time. In most cases this will not affect the repayment amount but the loan will be repaid quicker if the interest rate falls, or over a longer period if the rate increases.

Banks traditionally view pharmacies as they do any other retail outlet and have traditionally ignored the value of the NHS contract and the general resilience of prescription turnover in recessionary periods. This situation led to the emergence of loan schemes to facilitate the process by which pharmacists could borrow money at favourable rates.

Loan schemes have been developed by wholesalers, anxious to maintain their share of the wholesale market. The wholesaler does not supply the funds but merely facilitates the availability of funds and acts as security for the money. The arrangement fee is usually higher than the bank arrangement fee and cannot be negotiated. It might be as high as 2% of the loan. The most single voiced criticism of loan schemes operated by wholesalers is the stipulation that 70% of all goods should be bought from them. Again, you will be required to fund about 20% of the project from your own funds.

Unichem was the first company to set up a scheme and a number of pharmacists have bought their pharmacies through this scheme.

Building societies are becoming interested in funding business and might be a considered option. They may advise you to take out an endowment policy and only the interest is repaid. You should be very cautious with this approach as it is not attractive to business. The endowment premium is not allowable against tax as it is regarded by HM Inspector of Taxes (HMIT) as a savings policy. You should also be cautious since in recent years some endowments have not been performing very well. This problem has occurred due to low inflation and low interest. In some cases endowments have not made sufficient money to pay off the enterprise they were designed for.

QUESTION 11: ASSESSING ACCOUNTS

I have obtained the accounts for a pharmacy (Tables 1–4) that I am intending to buy. Are there any simple calculations that I might perform that would improve the way I view the accounts?

Table 1 Profit and loss accounts

	1991	1992	1993
Sales NHS	145014	161618	158007
Counter	62149	69266	85071
Total sales	207163	230884	243078
Opening stock	26157	24110	27684
Purchases	138875	156268	169611
	165032	180378	197295
Closing stock	24110	27684	25725
Cost of sales	140922	152694	171570
Gross profit	66241	78190	71508
Expenses:			
Wages and NIC	9745	16057	29920
Rent and rates	5213	3234	1760
General insurance	1972	2583	880
Motor expenses	2955	4264	4049
Light and heat	1863	1586	1555
Telephone	1863	2414	1804
Replacement/renewal	456	1024	6049
Postage/advertising	1022	1413	1620
Professional subs	1253	1573	1537
Accountancy	412	360	540
General expenses	3513	2947	1851
Depreciation	3167	2762	3399
Locum fees	2425	1030	1760
TOTAL EXPENSES	35859	41247	56724
NET PROFIT	30382	36943	14784

Table 2 Balance sheet at 31 December 1991

	Forward	Addition	Dep.	NBV
Fixed assets:				
Motor car	5346	4854	(2040)	8160
Fixture and fittings	10032	1243	(1127)	10148
	15378	6097	(3167)	18308
Intangible assets:				
Goodwill at cost				8000
				26308
Current assets:				
Cash in hand				192
Cash at bank				776
Trade debtors/				
prepayment				24296
Stock in trade				24100
				49364
Current liabilities:				
Creditors and accruals				27150
Bank loan account				3888
Special advance from Health Authority				11400
				42438
Net current assets				6926
Net assets				£ 33234
Financed by capital account:				
Balance brought forward				23320
Add net profit				30382
Interest received				430
				54132
Deduct drawings				20898
				£ 33234

NBV = Net book value; Dep. = Depreciation

Table 3 Balance sheet at 31 December 1992

	Forward	Addition	Dep.	NBV
Fixed assets:				
Property purchase		31642		31642
Motor car	8160	–	(1632)	6528
Fixture and fittings	10148	1155	(1130)	10173
	18308	32797	(2762)	48343
Intangible assets:				
Goodwill at cost				8000
				56343
Current assets:				
Cash in hand				197
Trade debtors/				
prepayment				30672
Stock in trade				27684
				58553
Current liabilities:				
Bank overdraft				387
Bank loan account				26760
Creditors and accruals				42784
				69907
Net current assets				114896
Net assets				£ 44989
Financed by capital account:				
Balance brought forward (1991)				33234
Add net profit				36943
Deduct drawings				25212
				£ 44965

NBV = Net book value; Dep. = Depreciation

Table 4 Balance sheet at 31 December 1993

	Forward	Addition	Dep.	NBV
Fixed assets:				
Property	31642	7488	–	39130
Motor car	6528	–	(1306)	5222
Fixture and fittings	10173	10760	(2093)	18804
	48343	18248	(3399)	63156
Current assets:				
Cash in hand				116
Trade debtors/				
prepayment				40078
Stock in trade				25725
				65919
Current liabilities:				
Bank overdraft				6388
Bank loan account				40963
Creditors and accruals				12300
				59651
Net current assets				6268
Net assets				£ 69424
Financed by capital account:				
Balance brought forward (1992)				44965
Add net profit				14784
				59749
Deduct drawings				11193
Goodwill written off				8000
				19049
				£ 40700

NBV = Net book value; Dep. = Depreciation

ANSWER

By calculating a number of ratios you can see more clearly how the business is performing. This has been done in Table 5. The analysis improves the precision with which the accounts can be viewed. Some of the terms may need further explanation. 'Average stock' (line 5) is the mean of the opening and closing stock. 'Manager's salary'(line 15) is the salary the pharmacist might hope to earn if he was employed by someone else. For the purpose of this exercise, the figure should be increased by £1000 per year. In 1993 the pharmacist employed a full-time pharmacist – note the rise in wages. This therefore reduced the notional salary. Line 16 includes the manager's salary (line 15) in the total wages bill. The implication of the manager's salary is that the real net profit line is actually less than shown in the profit and loss account. 'Capital employed' (line 20) equates to the net assets in the balance sheet.

Taking goodwill (line 22) and deducting the £8000 goodwill the pharmacist paid in 1986, gives a clearer picture of what return is being generated from the real value of the business.

In short, if the pharmacist was to sell the business tomorrow would he be better off getting a job for £20 000 per annum and employing the capital elsewhere, e.g. inserting it in a high interest deposit account or into stocks and shares?

In this business clearly he would be well advised to stay put. The return on capital, even when considering the real capital value of the business, is on average 11.26% over the three years shown. Few investments would produce this degree of return. Additionally, you have the luxury of running your own business.

Table 5 Viewing the accounts

Year ending 31 December 1990	1991	1992	1993
1 Turnover (£)	207163	230884	243078
2 Gross profit (£)	66241	78190	71508
3 Gross margin % (2/1)	31.9%	33.86%	29.41%
4 Cost of goods sold (£)	140922	152694	171570
5 Average stock (£)	25133	25897	26704.50
6 Stockturn (4/5)	5.6	5.8	6.4
7 Stockturn (end stock)	5.8	5.51	6.7
8 Stockturn (end stock & 1)	8.6	8.34	9.4
9 Expenses (£)	35859	41247	56724
10 Expenses % turnover	17.3%	17.8%	23.3%
11 Wages (3)	9745	16057	29920
12 Wages % turnover	4.7%	6.9%	12.3%
13 Net operating profit	30382	36943	14784
14 NOP as % turnover	14.7%	16.0%	6.1%
15 Manager's salary estimate* (£)	21000	22000	10000
16 Total wages	30745	38057	39920
17 Total wages % turnover	14.8%	16.5%	16.4%
18 Real net profit (13–15)	9382	14943	4784
19 RNP as % of turnover	4.5%	6.5%	2.0%
20 Capital employed**	33234	44965	40700
21 Return on capital % (18/20)	28%	33%	11.7%
22 Goodwill (5 × line 18)	46910	74715	23920
23 Capital employed + line 22	80144	119680	64620
24 Return on capital % (18/23)	11.7%	12.48%	7.4%

*   In 1993 manager's salary is estimated at £10 000 since the owner
employed a full-time pharmacy manager.
** Capital employed refers to the bottom line of the balance sheet for
that year.

QUESTION 12: LIMITED LIABILITY COMPANY

I am in the process of buying a pharmacy which is a limited company. Should I retain the limited company status or should I trade as a sole trader?

ANSWER

The advice from most accountants would be that you should avoid the limited company status and simply buy the assets of the company. There is no tax advantage to you from being a limited company and, since you will be required to have fully audited accounts each year, the cost of compiling accounts for a limited company might be double what you would pay to have your accounts compiled as a sole trader. Your accounts must be registered with Companies House and will be available for public scrutiny. Failure to submit accounts on time will attract a fine.

If you are undertaking a high risk venture you might wish to protect yourself and in such circumstances you may consider having a limited liability company which is designed to limit the liability you have in the case where it fails. However, limited liability only covers you so far. If you are found to be acting illegally then your liability is removed. For example, if it could be proved that you were carrying on the business and trading at a time when you knew that the business was insolvent then you could personally be liable for losses.

Banks will lend money to limited companies but they will often require personal guarantees from you and you can, for example, lose your home if the business fails.

A limited company is an independent legal entity. If you decide to take on the company you must indemnify yourself against any undisclosed liabilities that the company may be responsible for, such as unpaid VAT and PAYE.

Questions 13–16 relate to the pharmacy whose accounts are given in Tables 1–4.

QUESTION 13: GROSS PROFIT

I have been keen to purchase a pharmacy and have approached the owner who is in his early 50s. He has asked his accountant to supply me with the last three years' accounts (Tables 1–4). These seem to be in order except that last year there was approximately a 4% drop in gross profit. What reasons might there be for such a sharp drop in profit?

ANSWER

The 1993 profit and loss accounts show a fall in gross profit compared to 1992 in spite of an increase in turnover. This situation generally arises for two reasons: (a) competition – having to lower the profit margin; and (b) product mix – selling more products that have a low profit margin, e.g. nappies. The main explanation is a fall in profitability from Health Service prescriptions. This pharmacy generates 70% of its turnover from Health Service dispensing and, in common with all UK pharmacies, the business had experienced a drop in gross profit from this source in 1993. Comparing the percentage gross profit for 1991, 1992 and 1993 we find it to be 31.9%, 33.8% and 29.4% respectively. The 4.4% change in gross margin between 1992 and 1993 represents £10 580 less gross profit. The accountant is, understandably, concerned that you explain this fully. He is not satisfied that the fall in NHS gross profit is sufficient to explain the 1992 to 1993 drop. He will then consider other issues that affect gross profit. The profit margin shown on these accounts is high.

In 1992 the pharmacy supplied oxygen to five patients, in 1993 it supplied none. Oxygen is a very profitable aspect of dispensing taking into account the additional fees payable. This can be used to explain part of the 4.4% differential in gross profit.

The average community pharmacy might have a profit margin of 24% and some, particularly if they have very large numbers of prescriptions, might have a profit margin as low as 15%.

QUESTION 14: PRICING POLICY

What can be the effect of a change in pricing policy for the business?

ANSWER

In late 1993 a Superdrug store opened within walking distance from the pharmacy. The pharmacist, anticipating the competition decided to have a 'sale'. He cut the price of his nappies to near cost price for one month and a further 10% off all baby goods. This increased customer flow but reduced gross profit.

You will need to consider if a further reduction on counter margins will be necessary to compete effectively with the newly established Superdrug store. This will have implications for your projected cash-flow figures.

QUESTION 15: STOCKHOLDING

There has been a considerable reduction in stockholding. What would have allowed this to happen?

ANSWER

The pharmacy has had a major refit and this has included a reduction in the amount of store space and a smaller dispensary. This has allowed a more efficient stock level and it is doubtful if you could make additional reduction if you take over the business. So efficiencies in this area are limited and would not be a major feature of your business plan to the bank.

QUESTION 16: REASONS FOR SELLING A PHARMACY

I am very keen to buy this business. I hope that my urgency does not cloud my objectivity. Are there any basic questions I should be asking?

ANSWER

Yes. 'Why is this pharmacist selling his business?', would be a good one. The pharmacist is in his mid-40s and is selling the business after investing heavily in recent years and you must ask why he now wishes to sell. At his age selling will not provide any retirement relief from tax. Is there something wrong with the business? You may find that his reason is personal. For example, he or his wife is ill and this has prompted him to retire. There is no age limit to when you can retire from employment.

Not identifying a genuine reason for selling must be viewed with suspicion. Perhaps a new shopping centre is planned that will severely affect the business or the local GPs might have decided to relocate their practice.

QUESTION 17: BANK LOAN INTEREST

I have just agreed the purchase of a pharmacy and have got most of the money from the bank as a loan. The rate of interest is 2% above base which I am told is a good rate. What does this mean?

ANSWER

If the base rate is 7% and you are required to pay 2% above base rate, then your rate of interest will be 9% on your loan. The base rate is set by the banks, but it is heavily influenced by the Bank of England which effectively determines the rate.

As you know there are often changes in the base rate of interest. This is usually due to the Government responding to changes in the economy. The Government may wish to stimulate growth by lowering the base rate or encourage people to save by increasing it.

Your interest therefore may change over the period of your loan and this could cause severe cash-flow problems. If this occurs and you find that your interest repayments have increased you might consider going back to your bank manager to renegotiate the repayment over a longer period of time. In essence you keep the same rate of repayment but pay it over a longer period.

QUESTION 18: PERSONAL MONIES INTRODUCED

Apart from the bank loan my parents have given me £35 000 towards the purchase of my pharmacy and I have £10 000 of my own savings. Will I be taxed on the money I use to purchase the business?

ANSWER

The bank loan is typically paid back over seven to ten years and tax relief is available on the interest paid on this loan. You will not normally be taxed on personal savings or 'gifts' of money. You will have paid your tax on your savings. Money 'gifted', for example from a parent, will be subject to the inheritance tax rules. This is a complex area and you must obtain tax advice on any money gifted. For example, tax may be due on the gift if the grantor dies within seven years of making it.

QUESTION 19: FIXTURES AND FITTINGS

I am keen to make an offer for a pharmacy. What should I pay for fixtures and fittings and goodwill?

ANSWER

Fixtures and fittings will be written off by depreciation over an agreed period, usually ten years, and you can make claims against tax for this depreciation. Goodwill is usually written off but this cannot be claimed against tax.

Goodwill is an intangible asset representing the benefit for the purchaser to obtain future earnings from the established business. It is a difficult item to value and is ultimately determined by the market. One method of estimating the goodwill of any business is to multiply real net profit (RNP) by three to five (see Table 5). It is accepted that, if a new business opens, it would take three to five years to become as popular as an existing business. Since limitation of dispensing contacts remains, pharmacies are obtaining premium prices and you would therefore be justified in estimating the maximum goodwill value of five years – in some cases this might be conservative.

Running a pharmacy

When reps are discussing bonus deals with me they always refer to profit and I am never clear how I might calculate this. Can you explain?

ANSWER

Profit, as a percentage, will depend on whether it is profit on the cost of the item or on the sale price of the item – profit on return (POR). Reps will often refer to profit as profit on cost rather than POR. From a business point of view you should be judging the merits of a bonus deal on POR.

    Let us consider a bottle of cough medicine that has a retail price of £2.00 and a trade price (excl. VAT) of £1.00. You must first establish the retail price without VAT as the VAT is not yours and must be paid to Customs and Excise. You calculate the VAT component (17.5%) of a retail price by multiplying it by seven and dividing it by 47.

    £2.00 contains 30p of VAT
    Selling price excl. VAT (return) is £1.70
    Profit is 70p
    POR is 41%
    Profit on cost is 70%.

A rep. who tells you that you make 70% profit is misrepresenting the benefit to your business of buying his deal.

QUESTION 21: PART-TIME EMPLOYEES

I have been notified that I will be having a visit from an inspector from the local social security office. He wishes to inspect all my records on staff salaries including the records of part-time staff. I have been keeping P11 worksheets for my part-time staff. Is this incorrect?

ANSWER

Yes. A business is required to operate PAYE for each employee including those who do not earn enough to pay Income Tax or National Insurance Contributions (NICs). Currently, employees who are paid £57.99 or less will not pay NICs. The position of a locum pharmacist has caused particular problems in recent years. A regular locum must be regarded as an employee and indeed it is suggested that an occasional locum, unless he/she has a tax exemption certificate issued by the local tax office, must be considered for PAYE.

When you pay an employee you must calculate his/her tax and NIC, make any necessary deductions and make a record on the P11 worksheets provided by the Inland Revenue for that employee. If no deductions are due you are still required to note the payment made. Additionally, you are required to supply employees with notification of what deductions have been made. This is usually a written statement on their pay-slip. It is required by law to prepare a pay-slip for each salary payment.

For part-time employees you must also have a P46 form signed by them declaring that this is their only job.

QUESTION 22: PAYE TAX CODES

I have been using the emergency tax code – currently 352L – for all my employees. One of my female members of staff is over 60 and, although I

have not been informed officially, is claiming a state pension. Will I still be
required to keep records of her pay now that she has retired?

ANSWER

Yes. She is not retired as such since she is still in employment and is simply drawing her pension which she is entitled to do. Her pension is taxable income. You will need to write to your local tax inspector and give details. He will then amend the employee's code to take account of her pension. If she was a part-time employee then her P46 form that declared her to have no other salary source is no longer valid.

QUESTION 23: PAYE

I have just started a business and have one full-time member of staff and
two part-time members of staff. When and how should I pay their tax and
NIC?

ANSWER

You will need to inform HM Inspector of Taxes (HMIT) at your local tax office that you have set up in business. They will send all relevant forms, set up an account and send you a pay book so that you can pay in any payments.

Within 14 days after the end of the month in which a wage was paid, you are required to pay any tax and NIC due to the Inland Revenue and payment forms are provided for this purpose.

At the end of the tax year, 5 April, you are required to provide your local tax office with a completed P35 form within 14 days. This form indicates the tax and NIC you have paid for each employee during the year. You must also supply the names of employees for whom you did not pay tax.

You must provide each employee who pays tax with a P60 form which is a statement of the tax and NIC you have paid on their behalf.

If an employee leaves your employment during the year you are required to supply them with a P45 form. This is a statement of how much tax they have paid to date and it can be used by their next employer to insert them onto a P11 form at the appropriate week. Part of the P45 form must be sent to your local tax office on the date the employee leaves.

QUESTION 24: PREGNANT EMPLOYEE

One of my full-time employees has just announced that she is pregnant. She has been with me for four months and, although I believe she knew she was expecting when she accepted the job, she did not inform me of this. Can I dismiss her for concealing this information?

ANSWER

No. If you dismiss her you will most probably be facing a case for unfair dismissal. You are required to pay statutory maternity pay (SMP) to any employee who is in continuous employment for a period of at least 26 weeks and this period must include at least one day in the qualifying week (15th week before the week in which the baby is due, i.e. the employee's 26th week of pregnancy). However, they must be earning at least enough to pay NICs. Those not eligible to receive SMP include self-employed persons since they do not pay Class 1 National Insurance if the baby is stillborn before 29 weeks of pregnancy, if the person is taken into legal custody or if the employee goes abroad outside the EEC. You must be informed by the employee of the date on which the baby is due and be given at least 21 days' notice of the date she intends to stop work to have the baby. This notification can be requested in writing.

QUESTION 25: STATUTORY MATERNITY PAY

What amount of SMP am I required to pay and what records must be kept? More importantly, can I recover it?

ANSWER

Statutory maternity pay can be paid for a period of up to 18 weeks – the maternity pay period. The employee can get SMP from the beginning of the 11th week before the week in which the baby is due (from the Sunday of the 30th week of pregnancy). The pay can only be made if the employee has stopped work. It is up to the employee how long she wishes to remain at work so long as the pregnancy is not preventing her from doing the job properly. Dismissal because of pregnancy may in some cases be deemed fair if the employee is unable to do the job or if the job might be dangerous for the employee.

As long as the employee stops before the 6th week before the week in which the baby is due she is entitled to receive SMP for the full 18-week period. If she decides to work longer she will lose the SMP payment for each week in which she worked.

The amount of SMP paid depends on the length of employment and how much the employee is paid. The standard rate is paid to all employees who qualify and is a flat rate payment which is £47.95 in 1995–6. A higher rate is paid for the first six weeks of the 18-week period to those employees who have been continuously employed for at least two years full-time or five years part-time. Part-time means employed for less than 16 hours per week. The higher rate payment is 90% of the employee's weekly earnings and will never be lower than the lower rate.

SMP is paid at the same time as wages. It must be treated as income in the same way as wages and therefore a record kept of the payment made in the PAYE worksheet P11. You can recover SMP from NIC.

QUESTION 26: CONTINUATION OF EMPLOYMENT

I have taken over a pharmacy and along with it the staff. When one member of staff was off ill for a week recently I paid her statutory sick pay (SSP). She now informs me that she has a right to have her full pay as her previous employer paid her full pay while on sick leave. What is the basis of her claim?

ANSWER

One of the difficulties of retaining staff when taking over a business is that you also take over the contract that they had with the previous employer. If the previous employer as a matter of routine paid staff their full pay during short periods of illness they would claim that you must continue this precedent and this is likely to be the opinion of an industrial tribunal.

You should have a new contract of employment with them setting out your terms of employment. If they sign this it may dissuade them from taking a claim for unfair dismissal.

QUESTION 27: STATUTORY SICK PAY

So I am liable to pay her full pay. Can I therefore treat this payment as SSP and make claims based on it?

ANSWER

Any agreement you make – or in this case are forced into – to pay full pay during sickness is between you and the employee. SSP can only apply to the amount that has been identified by the Government which is £52.50 per week in 1995–6 for days that qualify for SSP. It cannot be paid unless the employee is sick for at least four days in a row. All days count, including weekends, holidays and days off. The first three days of a sickness spell are termed waiting days. Any days of sickness after that will be regarded as qualifying days. SSP is paid only for qualifying days and these include the days of the week they are employed to work, e.g. Monday to Friday. If it is less than eight weeks since the employee was sick for four or more days in a row, three waiting days are not required before SSP is paid. Qualifying days taken up to eight weeks earlier can count as waiting days for the next spell of sickness. This is because any spells of sickness of four or more days in a row with less than eight weeks between them are linked. The start of the linked period of sickness is the beginning of the first of the spells that link together, but linked periods can only be allowed if they happen in the same employment.

Employees are required to inform you that they are unable to come to work because they are ill. This should be outlined in the staff handbook which each employee should have received. You might also state in the handbook what evidence of illness you require. When an employee is sick for less than seven days, you might require him/her to complete a self-certificate form (form SC2). If he/she is sick for more than seven days, you can request the employee to provide medical evidence that he/she is sick.

SSP is paid by you at the relevant rate and it must be treated as income and therefore might be subject to tax and NIC. By making the necessary records the employer may be able to reclaim some of the SSP that has been paid in the tax month (see Question 28). In some smaller businesses however, the NIC paid by other employees might not be enough to recoup SSP. In such situations the SSP may be recouped from the tax. In the very rare event of this not being enough you will need to apply in writing to the DHSS for a refund.

A form is available to record SSP which should identify waiting days and qualifying days. Additionally, a record of SSP paid should be included on the PAYE P11 worksheet and in the cash book.

To be eligible for SSP the employee must have earned enough to have paid NIC. Two rates of SSP are payable and which rate applies will depend on how much the employee earned before becoming sick. SSP is paid by the employee for 28 weeks in any sickness spell. At that time, if the employee remains ill he/she will then claim benefit from the Social Services (DHSS in Northern Ireland).

QUESTION 28: CLAIMING BACK SSP

Will I be able to claim back the SSP I pay out to employees who are ill?

ANSWER

Maybe but possibly not a lot. Before 1994 the SSP small employers' relief scheme allowed employers to claim back SSP. After 1994 it was replaced by the Percentage Threshold Scheme. The Percentage Threshold Scheme is designed to help employers who have a high proportion of their workforce sick at one time. Under the new scheme you must compare the total SSP you have paid in a tax month with 13% of your total, employer's and employees gross Class 1 NICs for the tax month. The scheme appears involved but basically this is how it operates.

Work out the total gross Class 1 NIC liability for the tax month. Multiply this by 0.13 (13%) – call this amount A. Next work out the total SSP for that month – call this amount B. You can recover the amount that B exceeds A.

Your SSP for the month was £110.00
13% of your Class 1 NIC works out at £120.00
You would be able to recover £10.00 of SSP.

You would then deduct the amount that you are expected to recover from the payments you make to the Inland Revenue.

QUESTION 29: CLAIMING BACK SMP

I have heard that I will probably no longer be able to reclaim SSP, but does this also mean that I will not be able to reclaim SMP?

ANSWER

No. Like the rules governing payment of SSP, the rules governing SMP changed in 1994. Since then, if an employer does not qualify for Small

Employers' Relief, they can only recover 92% of the SMP they have paid to their employees. Those that qualify for Small Employers' Relief can recover 100% of the SMP that they have paid out and 5% compensation.

An employer who qualifies for Small Employers' Relief is someone who paid Class 1 NICs of £20000 or less in the qualifying tax year. The qualifying tax year refers to the last complete tax year before the pregnant employee's qualifying week.

If you were an employer for less than 12 months you would be allowed to estimate if you are eligible for Small Employers' Relief. Add your total Class 1 NICs due in the year and divide by the number of months you were an employer then multiply by 12. If this amount is £20000 or less you will qualify.

You should deduct the amount you are entitled to recover from your payments to the Inland Revenue and you do not need to make a special entry.

QUESTION 30: VALUE ADDED TAX (VAT)

I have just opened a VAT account and have received a VAT number. According to the information and instructions I am expected to wait for three months to reclaim back the VAT I have paid out on the drugs that I have purchased. This is going to severely affect my cash flow. Is there anything I can do?

ANSWER

Yes, Customs and Excise will allow you to reclaim your VAT monthly and you must apply in writing to get this concession explaining that you are experiencing cash flow problems. Pharmacies, as with all other businesses, are required by law to undertake assessment of their VAT liability – usually every three months. However, pharmacies, along with butchers, are unique among traders in that they usually receive repayments from Customs and Excise.

Each business that is registered for VAT must make returns quarterly. Pharmacies are allowed to do this monthly since they will be claiming VAT back and this is necessary for cash-flow purposes. A form is sent to the pharmacy and indicates the date by which the completed form must be returned.

QUESTION 31: VAT EXPLAINED

I find VAT very confusing. Is there a simple way to explain what it is and how I can manage it better within my business?

ANSWER

VAT is a purchase tax, a levy charged by the Government on someone purchasing an item or a service. There are two rates of VAT in the UK, zero rate (0%) – foods and children's clothing, and standard rate – 17.5% in 1995–6. Some items and services do not attract VAT, e.g. package holidays are classified as exempt. Only customers pay VAT, businesses do not pay VAT. Businesses do, however, have a statutory responsibility to collect VAT on behalf of the Government. Businesses of a certain nature, e.g. travel agencies or those having a low annual turnover – less than £46 000 per year – might wish not to be registered for VAT. However, there are certain advantages from registration in that VAT charged to the business for services used by the business, i.e. builders or shopfitters, may be reclaimed.

When a VAT registered business supplies goods or a service to another VAT registered business, the supplying business is obliged to provide a VAT invoice for each transaction indicating: (a) the supplier's name and address with VAT registration number; (b) the customer's name and address; (c) the date; (d) the invoice number (unique); (e) the total value of the invoice; (f) amount of zero-rated goods; and (g) VAT at the appropriate rate.

Take the example of a clock manufacturer who produces a clock and wishes to charge the wholesaler £50 for it. The manufacturer will write a VAT invoice for £50 plus £8.75 VAT, for a total of £58.75. This £58.75 will be paid to the manufacturer by the wholesaler at the end of the agreed credit period. At the end of the quarter in which the transaction took place, the manufacturer will make a VAT return to Customs and Excise and in it will pay the £8.75 due to the manufacturer for the clock.

The wholesaler will sell the clock on to a retailer for £100, making 50% profit on return, and will create a VAT invoice for £100 plus £17.50 – a total invoice of £117.50. At the end of the agreed credit period the retailer will pay the wholesaler £117.50. At the end of the quarter in which the transaction took place the wholesaler will make a VAT return in which he will pay Customs and Excise £8.75 of the £17.50 VAT which is due since he has already paid £8.75 of the VAT due on the clock when paying the wholesaler. You will remember that the wholesaler has already paid £8.75 of the VAT due when paying the manufacturer.

The retailer will sell the clock to a customer for £200 making 100% profit and will be obliged to add on £35 VAT. Since the customer will be responsible for paying VAT there is no need to identify the VAT element of the price on the receipt for £235. Where the customer is a foreign visitor buying the clock for use outside the UK, the customer can claim back the VAT on leaving the country. At the end of the quarter in which the transaction took place the retailer will pay Customs and Excise £17.50 of the VAT due on the clock. He has already paid £17.50 when paying the wholesaler's bill.

The net effect of this process is that Customs and Excise has collected the exact amount of VAT due on the clock when it is sold without knowing what the final retail price was.

QUESTION 32: VAT – ZERO-RATED GOODS

I have always used scheme B for calculation of my VAT. As a rule of thumb I usually multiply all my zero-rated goods by a factor of 1.5 to calculate the zero rate uplift value. Will this be acceptable to Customs and Excise?

ANSWER

If you can justify it as correct and can show that it is an effective way of calculating what VAT you owe then it will be acceptable. However, you must be sure that if you receive an inspection this figure measures up. For example, the VAT inspector will look at the retail price you have for a number of zero-rated items such as nappies and baby milks and compare how their sale price measures up to your estimated uplift.

In addition he will look for zero-rated items that have been dispensed on prescription and check that you have not put them through your business as if they were sold via the till. Such items might include specialized foods for coeliac disease, phenylketonuria and milk sensitivity. You must be very clear on which items are zero-rated and which are not.

QUESTION 33: VAT – MAKING RETURNS

Until recently I had my VAT return processed by my accountant. I now find this too expensive and wish to do the return myself. Can you give me an overview of what is involved?

ANSWER

There are two areas where money enters the business:

1 money paid by Health Authorities (CSA in Northern Ireland and Health Boards in Scotland) for NHS prescriptions dispensed; and
2 money collected at the till for counter sales including over-the-counter (OTC) medicines.

Medicines dispensed on a doctor's prescription are zero-rated. Medicine supplied by other sources, e.g. sold OTC or on a stock prescription from a GP, are subject to VAT at the standard rate. Pharmacies will have paid VAT to the wholesaler for all medicines received but the monies paid to pharmacies by Health Authorities (CSA in Northern Ireland and Health Boards in Scotland) does not include VAT.

All goods sold OTC will be subject to VAT at the appropriate rate. This VAT will be due to Customs and Excise at the end of the quarter in which the transaction took place. Therefore, from the prescriptions dispensed the pharmacy will be owed VAT but will owe VAT from counter sales. It would be very difficult to identify how much VAT must be paid on each item sold and therefore a scheme for calculation of VAT liability is used to simplify the calculation. The scheme that best suits a community pharmacy is scheme B since we deal with two rates of VAT.

The VAT liability of the pharmacy is calculated from: (a) records of all invoices received; (b) total sales at the till; and (c) money received for dispensing NHS prescriptions.

All invoices received are recorded on a table such as Table 6. They may be recorded more easily on a database or spreadsheet program on a computer.

Table 6 Details recorded on invoices received in the pharmacy

Date	Supplier	Amount	VAT	Zero rate	Zero uplift
14/12/94	Sangers	69.10	0.79	63.7	87.00
15/12/94	AAH	117.50	17.50	0.00	0.00
16/12/94	Swains	21.09	3.14	0.00	0.00

At the end of the month summing each of the columns in Table 6 will give the total paid out to wholesalers and other suppliers, total VAT paid and total of zero-rated goods received. The zero-rated uplift refers to the value that this item will sell for. The VAT is calculated from the total till takings minus the total zero rate uplift value.

Shop sales are registered at the till. By totalling all sales we can calculate the amount of VAT collected. The zero-rated goods sold are calculated from the invoices and the sum of the zero rate uplift items that were sold via the till are deducted from the total till receipts for the month. The VAT due is then calculated by multiplying by seven and dividing by 47.

Consider this example:

Till receipts for the month	£4000
Sum of zero rate uplift for month	£1000
Money on which VAT is due	£3000
7/47ths of £3000 (VAT due)	£446.80

You can check if you are correct by taking £446.80 from £3000 to give £2553.20. Calculating 17.5% of this figure gives £446.80 – the VAT due.

QUESTION 34: VAT – ZERO-RATED ITEMS

I understand that a number of items that are not normally zero-rated can become zero-rated when sold in a pharmacy. Can you advise?

ANSWER

The VAT status of an item may change due to the circumstances of the sale. The simplest example is anything that is dispensed as a private prescription for a human will be exempt from VAT. This does not apply to prescriptions for treating animals. Nicotine replacement therapy patches and gum cannot be sold OTC to a pregnant or diabetic patient. However, a GP may write a private prescription by which they may then buy them. In such cases the cost is free of VAT.

Medical devices such as glucose meters and nebulizers, when used in the management of a patient's condition, will be exempt from VAT. To get this exemption you will need to obtain a declaration either from the patient's doctor or the patient himself stating that the device is for the management of disease. This will allow you to reclaim the VAT you paid when purchasing the device from the supplier. The declaration must be kept for inspection by Customs and Excise.

Pregnancy tests performed in the pharmacy are also exempt from VAT. This exemption is included in Group 7 of VATA 1994 exemptions.

Customs and Excise keep the VAT status of a number of items under review. Such items are usually food products, e.g. olive oil.

QUESTION 35: VAT ON LOCUM FEES

I own my own pharmacy and I am registered for VAT. On reading the VAT regulations, I understand that if I provide a service in most cases I must charge VAT. My pharmacy is open Monday to Friday and occasionally on Saturday I may do a locum for a colleague. Should I be charging VAT?

ANSWER

No. Locum fees for providing pharmaceutical services are exempt from VAT. But you are correct in that on any other service you provide you should be paying VAT. For example, if you acted as a consultant to a Health Authority or a pharmaceutical company then you would be required to provide them with an invoice and you must charge VAT at the standard rate of 17.5%.

QUESTION 36: MEALS AS BUSINESS EXPENSES

I have just entertained the manager of the local residential home to lunch. Last year my accountant told me that I could claim the staff Christmas dinner as an expense. Can I claim this expense against tax since it has ensured that we continue to provide our services to the home?

ANSWER

No. Entertainment of this kind is not allowable against tax even though it may seem a business activity. You are allowed to claim the staff Christmas dinner, up to a cost of £75.00 per head, as a business expense as this is regarded as looking after your staff. You would be allowed to have staff members' spouses at the Christmas dinner and you would be allowed up to a cost of £50.00 for each of them. If you are forced to work late and require a member of staff to work with you, you could provide them with a meal and claim it as expenses.

QUESTION 37: STAFF CHRISTMAS BONUS

I give my staff a cash bonus of £200 each at Christmas. Do I need to include this on the P11 worksheets?

ANSWER

Yes. Your cash bonus is subject to National Insurance and Income Tax in exactly the same way as pay is. You would need to be careful since some members of staff who are not being paid enough to pay NIC or tax may be required to do so in the week that you give them their bonus.

QUESTION 38: STAFF REDUNDANCY

I have been forced to pay-off one of my long-serving full-time members of staff due to declining business. This has been a difficult affair. How can I calculate her redundancy and should it be treated for tax and PAYE?

ANSWER

The first thing you must do is to ensure that you do not become involved in an unfair dismissal case. To do this you must ensure that the redundancy has been 'fair'. Usually it would be deemed to be fair if it was the most junior member of staff – last in first out. This may not be possible since the saving from the wages of the senior member of staff is necessary for the business. Perhaps you might make a junior member of staff redundant and offer the senior member of staff the part-time post.

Redundancy only applies to members of staff who have been employed full-time for two years or part-time (up to 16 hours a week) for five years. They are normally paid one week's salary for each year of service. This scheme may now be changed in light of a legal case in September 1995 which showed that part-time employees should have the same rights as full-time employees.

Calculation of redundancy pay is not easy and is dependent on the number of years service. You would be best advised to contact your local Industrial Relations office for precise advice and the wording of all letters and agreements. As a general guide redundancy payments usually amount to one week's salary for each full year of service up to the age of 30. Between the ages of 30 and 50 it is two weeks' salary. Over 50 it will be more.

The redundancy payment is not treated as PAYE and is not included in the P11 worksheet. You will be required to give the employee a P45.

QUESTION 39: STAFF PURCHASES

I am concerned that some of my staff may not be paying for items which they claim they have purchased. Is there a standard procedure that I can implement to ensure that there is no confusion?

ANSWER

You have been imprudent not to have had a formalized procedure in place from the start. Staff pilfering is one of the greatest problems businesses have and this can adversely affect gross margins.

You should implement a procedure immediately. A staff purchase book must be put in place and all goods purchased by any member of staff must be recorded in the book along with the agreed staff discount. The pharmacist, or other senior member of staff, should also be charged with the responsibility of over-seeing the purchases, particularly the payment of monies. Money for staff purchases is best kept in a staff box and not rung into the till. This will allow you to reconcile the money in the staff box with the money in the staff book and will allow you to show your accountant how many goods were sold at discount.

A simple system like this will reduce any ambiguities or disputes that might arise when staff are found to be taking items from the premises. You may have difficulty implementing such a scheme as honest staff may feel they are being accused of dishonesty and dishonest staff will clearly not want it. You might sooth the implementation by claiming that your accountant requires this and you should ensure that all your own purchases are recorded in a similar way.

QUESTION 40: STAFF INTERVIEW

As an employer, I always feel that I do not get the best out of a job interview and I find it is not as effective as it should be. What should I be doing and what should I be aiming to achieve?

ANSWER

The interview is a very powerful selection method but is often misunderstood. Clearly the interview is designed to allow you, the prospective employer, an opportunity to meet and to assess in detail someone who will be employed in your business and who will be an asset to it. The interview is therefore not an opportunity to display your power or to impress upon a stranger how highly talented and successful you are.

First, be prepared. Have all details on job description, qualifications necessary, salary scale etc. Note any unclear or missing information that needs to be clarified and having checked the references be prepared to make comments on what previous employers have said.

An interview should be conducted in private without interruptions and, if possible, it should not be conducted from behind a desk. It should be relaxed and you should set the tone, establish control and state common goals of the interview process. This will ensure that the objective of the interview is met, namely that you obtain sufficient objective information about this candidate on which you can base a firm decision. The type of questions you ask will help. Open-ended questions will help to stimulate discussion and stop the candidate replying 'yes' or 'no'. However, one technique that scuppers more interviews is the use of the 'silence technique'. This means asking an open-ended question and then when the candidate has finished the reply leaving a silent pause. The usual response is that the candidate will feel they have to speak and will carry on to no avail.

For most jobs an interview should not be very long – a maximum of 30 to 45 minutes. Based on 30 minutes, an interview might be as follows:

- Introduction (five minutes) – This time should be used to reduce tension and 'break the ice' through friendly conversation. Additionally, you should confirm that you are familiar with the applicant's material and are prepared for the interview.
- Structure (one minute) – You should inform the applicant of how the interview will take place. For example: 'We will have the next 25 minutes to discuss the job and your qualifications. I will be asking you questions and taking notes. After that, you will have an opportunity to ask questions about the job and the company.'
- Body (15 minutes) – During this time you attempt to get a more complete picture of the applicant through the use of structured and unstructured questions and discussion. The purpose is to get the applicant to do most of the talking, this is their interview. As a rule of thumb you should talk for 20% of the time and they should talk for 80% of the time.
- Influence and sell (seven minutes) – You may feel that the candidate is very good and therefore there is a need to sell the company and why they should consider working for you.
- Summary (two minutes) – During the summary you should convey a positive feeling to the applicant. Allow questions to be asked and indicate when a decision will be made and how the applicant will be notified.

QUESTION 41: SEX DISCRIMINATION

I have been trying to employ a non-pharmacist manageress for one of my pharmacies. In the past three years I have employed two women who have left to have babies. Would it be reasonable to ask someone during the interview if she intends to add to her family?

ANSWER

Absolutely not. Even if the lady is not the most suitable for the job she would be in a position to sue for compensation for sex discrimination if you asked such a question. It is vitally important that you do not contravene employment laws relating to ethnic or sexual bias (also religious bias in Northern Ireland).

QUESTION 42: STAFF INDUCTION

When taking on a new member of staff what am I required to do?

ANSWER

There are two issues here. First, there are those things that you are required to do by law and there are those things that you should do to get the new member of staff off on the right footing. Start off as you intend to continue. Induction is training on day one but training should be a continuous process throughout the employment. Induction will also allow you to provide the employee with a contract of employment and start them on PAYE. Introduce them to the job and as a manager you should be personally involved while delegating induction tasks. Simple things such as a complete tour of the pharmacy and a warm and friendly approach will start the employee off with a positive feeling and a team approach.

A contract of employment must be given to each employee on starting a job or within 13 weeks. Without a written contract of employment, a contract still exists but the details will be heavily biased towards the employee should a dispute occur.

A staff handbook detailing disciplinary procedure may be appended to the contract and the employee, by signing the contract, will be familiar with these rules. This will include more details on use of the telephone, appropriate dress, absence and tardiness and purchasing articles in the pharmacy.

QUESTION 43: STOCK MANAGEMENT

I have found that my gross margin is considerably down this year and my accountant has asked me to review my purchasing procedure. He feels that my stock management is poor. What should I be looking at?

ANSWER

Stock management is an essential component of a successful and profitable business. Stock management means the controlling of goods when they are ordered, received, priced, stored, placed on sale, broken or damaged, pilfered, sold and returned for exchange or credit.

A system of management must be put in place to control each of these areas. The system employed must be simple to operate, practical, inexpensive and economical in terms of time, labour and materials, provide clear areas of responsibility and a quick clear picture of the situation so that action can be taken. Management in relation to stock control implies the need to control stock in addition to keeping it tidy and keeping detailed records. The system of stock control adopted should be based on efficient records of purchases and accurate physical stock counts from which sales can be calculated.

An electronic point of sale (EPOS) system is clearly the easiest way of doing this but it still requires a considerable amount of commitment.

QUESTION 44: STOCK TURNOVER RATIO

I appear to have too much stock for the turnover I am doing. It is not so clear where the overstock lies. What areas should I be looking at to get a reduction?

ANSWER

One of the aims of management will be to achieve a balance in the business to ensure that, as far as possible, the throughput of each section plays its proper part and that no one section is out of proportion to the others. Financial control should provide the manager with information on where profits and losses lie. This will require departmentalization. It is necessary to consider the purchases, sales and stockholding for each section separately, for only in this way can it be seen whether the proportion of stock held for any particular section is balanced with sales and whether the cost of stockholding for that section is justified by its profitability.

The basic aim of stock control therefore is to keep the stock tied up in unproductive stock as low as possible to free capital for more effective use.

Figures suggest that the average cost of stockholding can be as high as 26% of its value. This cost is made up from a number of factors – loss of interest on capital tied up in stock, the allocation of rent, rates and heating of stockroom area, the cost of maintaining the stockroom and keeping it tidy, losses through deterioration and breakages and the loss of productive capacity. You should remember that the greatest loss of potential profit occurs in the stockroom.

In general, the most important section in a pharmacy is the professional side of the business centred on the dispensary. Here special considerations apply and it is necessary to study the position carefully before attempting to apply general stock control methods. The stock of drugs and surgical dressings has to be adequate to meet demand on prescription. Stock control should help to keep the stock in perfect condition and in particular to avoid dead stock. Seasonal variation in the type of illness affects demand, as does the rapidly changing patterns of prescribing due to the introduction of new and more effective drugs. Demand depends therefore on a large number of variables outside the control of the pharmacist which acts against the ability for detailed stock control.

There is a stock control facility on most pharmacy computers which, using cumulative usage figures, estimates what should be held in stock to satisfy a month's demand.

The shopping area is logically divided up into sections, e.g. photographic, OTC medicines, health foods, baby-care etc. In this part of the pharmacy the demand for and range of stock offered for sale depends on the policy of the pharmacy and upon the demand from the public who use it. Information on sales from each section is essential.

By calculating the expected gross margin from the invoices it is possible, when the physical stock, the total purchases and the total sales are known, to calculate whether there has been any loss of goods by damage, pilferage or faulty checking of deliveries. This loss, the 'discrepancy' or 'shrinkage', is usually of the order of 1% in a well run business. In a business under management it should be watched particularly carefully. When such a system is in operation dishonesty and carelessness, such as errors in pricing, checking of deliveries etc. can be detected and the position rectified.

It follows that if detailed records of the whole business can be kept in this way it is possible, once statistics have been established, to institute a number of tight financial controls to help the manager forecast profits during the trading year. The assessment is, however, only a safe guide if careful stock control is kept to ensure that the figures obtained are accurate.

QUESTION 45: EPOS SYSTEM

I have been investigating the possibility of introducing an EPOS system but feel that the cost of buying the system is hard to justify as I am running an average-sized independent pharmacy.

ANSWER

The use of an EPOS system for stock control is by far the most efficient method of recording and analysing stock control. The system does demand considerable time at installation and time must be spent producing detailed analysis of data. I agree that it still remains expensive. An EPOS system will record stock levels as well as detailing purchases and will greatly increase your ability to manage your stock. Its main advantage is in maximizing stock efficiency – you can easily spot items that are not moving. It also appears to improve margins by ruling out incorrect pricing. On some occasions staff may price items incorrectly and whereas customers will complain about overpriced items, they will not complain about those which are underpriced.

Stock cards are a cheaper alternative. Their main disadvantage is the need to keep them up-to-date and in order. Due to the time involved in setting up a stock card index it is best to start initially with 20% of the fastest moving stock with an objective of covering the complete counter stock within one year. Stock cards are available from the National Pharmaceutical Association.

QUESTION 46: SHORT ITEMS OF STOCK

In an attempt to keep my stockholding under control I find that I am frequently running out of fast-moving items. How might I avoid this?

ANSWER

You must implement a stock control system that will record the stockholding and identify the minimum and maximum stockholding you need. The system must alert staff to reorder stock when the minimum stocking level is reached. There is a need to regularly update the stock level in light of identified trends. Trends will identify ups and downs in sales and allow the necessary action to be taken in revising stockholding. If it is found that a related product group is selling well, this is possibly an indication that the range of items should be increased. Conversely, if a group is selling well as a whole but the majority of sales are coming from one or two lines, the range probably could be reduced with advantage.

QUESTION 47: COST OF DISPLAY

A colleague has told me that he is thinking of getting rid of his baby food section as it is not profitable and does not justify the space that is allocated to it. How could I estimate the space I apportion to each section of my shop?

ANSWER

The value of display space can be estimated. For example, when considering a new line, you must decide if you can afford the display space that will be needed to obtain an adequate level of sales. A rough valuation of display space is given by the following equation.

$$\text{Cost (ft}^2\text{) of display} = \frac{\text{Area of display} \times \text{Fixed overheads}}{\text{Total sales area}}$$

In this equation, fixed overheads include light, heating, rent and rates. The only productive area of your shop is the sales area, therefore, the total fixed overheads must be applied to this area in square feet. Taking the idea further, some display areas are more valuable than others and a weighting can be applied, i.e. the till point is a very valuable area.

Since baby foods are traditionally low profit items you might find from this exercise that indeed it may be more sensible to do away with this line and replace it with, for example, a more profitable line such as food supplements.

QUESTION 48: OVER STOCKING

When a rep. is offering a bonus deal that appears to be attractive how can I gauge whether it will be of benefit to me?

ANSWER

Many offers, requiring you to buy a larger volume of stock than you would do normally, will be of benefit so long as you can sell all the stock efficiently. The total cost of an item falls with an increasing ordering quantity since purchasing costs will fall as bonuses are available. However, as a result of an increasing 'cost of stockholding' you eventually reach a point, 'the economic reordering quantity', after which the total cost rises. Therefore an attractive bonus offer may not always be best. For example the goods may go out of date. You may need to use your over-draft to pay for the goods which increases the real cost; and during storage goods may be damaged and some pilfered.

Unless a bonus parcel can be justified on a regular turnover basis, the order should not be placed. The only exception to the rule is where advertising or promotional activities on the part of the manufacturer fully justifies it.

QUESTION 49: STOCKTURN

What would be the ideal stockturn I should be aiming for?

ANSWER

Stockturn is the ratio obtained by dividing total sales at cost price by the average stock held at cost price. An annual stockturn for the whole business would ideally be set at eight, allowing for a six week stockholding. This is difficult to achieve. The cosmetic section of the average pharmacy causes the most difficult problem in stock control, particularly if the cosmetics are subject to agency agreements where a basic minimum stock has to be bought. Each stand will have slow moving lines. Critical assessment of a cosmetic agency line should be given particular consideration. It should ideally be turning over three to four times per year to be economically viable. Less than this and you might consider getting rid of it and replacing it with faster moving lines with the same profitability.

QUESTION 50: MARKETING IN PHARMACY

As a small retailer with two shops I have been in business for a number of years and know my customers. Are market principles really going to be of any benefit to me?

ANSWER

As a retailer you ignore the market at your peril. The most basic concept underlying marketing is that of human needs. A human need is a state of felt deprivation. It may be physical (food and medicines), social (belonging, affection) or individual (knowledge, self-expression).

A want is the form a human need takes based on culture or personality. Someone in the UK may want an aspirin to treat a headache whereas a Chinese person may want acupuncture. When needs and wants are backed up by buying power, wants become demands. Anything that can be offered for attention, acquisition, use, or consumption in order to satisfy wants or needs is called a product. The service a pharmacy offers is a product. Exchange occurs when someone satisfies a need or want by obtaining a product through offering something in return, usually money.

The world is a huge market place. In this market place people spend to satisfy needs and wants. Where a demand exists, someone will seek to supply what is needed – at a price. Where there is a substantial demand, many suppliers will be in competition to supply it. Those who do this well do so profitably and therefore acquire spending power, thus creating further demand.

The laws of supply and demand are by their nature unplanned. Essential needs may not be met since those in need may not have spending power. Additionally, some items that are demanded and supplied may not be socially desirable, e.g. illicit drugs. There is therefore a need for the State to regulate the market to some extent. This is called a 'mixed economy', a combination of market forces and central control.

QUESTION 51: COMPETING ON COST

A Superdrug store has just opened close to my pharmacy and they are very competitive. I have been attempting to cut my margins to compete but feel that in the long run this might be detrimental. Can you help?

ANSWER

Competition in the traditional pharmacy areas is increasing from non-pharmacy outlets. It can in some cases be financial suicide to attempt to take on giants like Superdrug on price alone as reduced margins will reduce, for example, your ability to keep up the appearance of your business. You should look at the areas in which they cannot compete, mainly the professional areas. You can give good quality advice which you might argue is not paid for but it does add to your goodwill and you are paid for it. More importantly find out what your customers want and supply it.

Marketing therefore is much more than a '50 pence off' offer on nappies. It includes everything about your business, from the assortment of goods and services offered to the decor and lighting, staff uniforms, staff attitude and customer care.

Consider this scenario which actually occurred in North London. A pharmacist decided to introduce a health food section in his pharmacy based on a need he had identified. Looking for space for this new section he found none was available. He then looked at items which he could possibly do away with. To his surprise a large section dedicated to disposable nappies was largely under-performing. He kept three major ranges of disposable nappy, Pampers, Togs and Peudouce. Recently a chain store had opened close by and was selling two of these ranges well below his selling price. Assessing customers, he noticed many coming into his shop having already purchased nappies. With nappies, price was the only element. He could not compete and make a profit. Removing the nappies and introducing health food improved his profit.

Market research is intended to complement experience, not replace it. If it confirms what you already suspected then you can act on knowledge confidently. However, the chances are that you will discover trends, requirements and competition of which you were unaware.

QUESTION 52: PHARMACY MISSION STATEMENT

Our local GP practice has a mission statement which they proudly display in the waiting room. What is the benefit of a mission statement and would we benefit from one?

ANSWER

A sense of mission is important for any organization and has obsessed American organizations over the last 20 years. Increasingly in the UK we are seeing companies with mission statements. Work in the 1950s identified the demise of the American railroad companies which came about because they viewed themselves as working in the railroad business, whereas they should have seen themselves in the transport business. If their mission had been stated as the latter they might not have suffered so severely from the trucking companies who took most of their traditional business.

A mission statement is important since it allows you to clearly select promotional methods and materials. Without a market-orientated mission statement pharmacists might spend money on promotions that do not focus on those consumer needs and wants that need to be satisfied. Promotion should be on strength and give the pharmacy a unique selling point.

A mission statement that one pharmacy has developed reads: 'To optimize our customers' health through the promotion of safe, effective and rational medicine use, provision of health advice and monitoring of disease within a profitable business enterprise.'

The advantage to the pharmacy is that it can clearly define the future. It would for example be keen to develop the sales of medical devices but not cut glass ornaments.

QUESTION 53: ADVERTISING COSTS

I have always been concerned with my pharmacy's image and have been considering more advertising. Is there any justification for a small pharmacy getting involved in advertising campaigns or is it money down the drain?

ANSWER

Telling people that you are there is not money down the drain but you must ensure that you use advertising money to get your message across effectively. There should be a consistent promotional message. With repeated exposure consumers will recognize them as having a common origin. If, for example, 'convenience' is to be promoted then this should be repeated in all promotional activities. Of course, the pharmacy should be convenient.

Many companies will spend about 1% of their turnover on advertising and promotion, while some very successful companies such as McDonalds will spend 13–16%.

Good promotion does not need to be expensive. Exchanging a friendly word with customers is very good promotion, your keenness to give friendly advice is the type of positive message that will be spread by word of mouth in close-knit communities. It is cheap and effective.

'All publicity is good publicity' is an adage that is definitely not true when it comes to small businesses. Just imagine seeing a newspaper story headlined, 'Restaurant fined for dirty kitchen', or even worse, 'Pharmacist fined'.

There may be an opportunity for free publicity in your local newspaper. They are interested in people and places and, contrary to public opinion, journalists do not spend their time chasing stories. Rather they sit and let the stories come to them. You might consider letting them know of any of your staff who has obtained a recent qualification. You might have a comment about the local traffic problem or the smoking policy on local public transport. All you need to do is create a positive public image which is consistent with the image you would like to project.

The biggest single advertisement is your pharmacy, which must speak loudly in marketing terms. Your pharmacy, especially the front of your shop, attracts customers and hopefully encourages them to pass through. Does your pharmacy have a modern recognizable facia? Does it suggest an old fashioned shop with old fashioned goods? Does it suggest bargain basement cut prices or high quality products? Is it attractive? Are window displays attractive and does it have a high standard of decor and maintenance? Take a walk outside and have a look. Are you happy with what you see?

QUESTION 54: MERCHANDISING

I am never sure if my pharmacy's layout is effective in ensuring the maximum number of sales. Is there a right and wrong way of setting things out?

ANSWER

Yes. Layout of a pharmacy is now a science and should not be ignored. A pharmacy should be designed to draw as many customers as possible past as much merchandise as possible. A successful layout will give 'four corner penetration'. The optimum design is rectangular with a 3:1 or 4:1 length to width ratio. High demand items such as OTC medicines and the dispensing department should be situated at the back. Clients should be drawn into the pharmacy along one aisle and exit by another aisle. Clearly a good design should take security into account.

The inside of the pharmacy should be visible from the street or shopping mall. It is known that people find it easier to enter a shop which they can see into compared to a shop where their view is restricted by a window display.

You should ensure that frequently used items are not all set on the same gondola but are distributed throughout the shop. For example, you might note that in your pharmacy, the best selling items are nappies, blades, medicines and deodorants. Ensuring that these items are not located together will mean that more clients will pass more of the products on display. It is important to get your customers to 'shop the shop'.

To appreciate the importance of merchandising consider the following research findings:

- 90% of pharmacy sales occur without the assistance of pharmacy staff
- 40% of buying decisions are made in the pharmacy
- 28% of first-time product purchasers see the product on display.

Good merchandising will sell more products.

QUESTION 55: STAFFING LEVELS

I feel that either I am over-staffed or under-staffed. How can I ensure that I have the right number of staff at all times?

ANSWER

Manpower planning is the first step in ensuring you have the right number of the right kind of employees. Where a new pharmacy is to be opened it is necessary to estimate the number and types of jobs that need filling immediately and at some future point. This will be based on your financial projections for a new pharmacy. In an existing pharmacy you should constantly review your manpower situation. Do you have enough staff? Do you have too many? Are any changes coming around, e.g. has a female employee just announced she is pregnant and will be going on maternity leave in three months? Manpower planning will ensure that you are not responding to crises which will only lead you to employing employees of a lesser quality than you would prefer.

It is difficult to create an equation for the most efficient complement of staff. In a smaller pharmacy you will know instinctively what staffing levels you require. Some larger businesses will set a limit of 3% to 5% of turnover for staff wages and this would be reviewed monthly. If the turnover is increasing then the manager could employ more part-time staff and if the turnover is falling his budget would require him to lay off some staff. A minimum wage for staff is agreed by the Joint Industrial Council (JIC) and information on the present rates is available from the National Pharmaceutical Association (NPA).

QUESTION 56: STAFFING LEVELS II

As an employer am I required to give my staff a written job description?

ANSWER

No. You are only required by law to give a contract of employment within 13 weeks of the employee starting the job. A job description is essential so that the employee and the manager knows what is to be done and from the initiation of any employment there is no confusion as to the employee's responsibilities. A good job description can only be written after a job analysis. To perform a job analysis you might observe a current employee doing the job, you might get them to complete a questionnaire if there are many undertaking a similar job or you might sit down with an employee and interview him/her on the job being performed.

The job description should include salary and annual incremental details as well as to whom the person is responsible and who, if anyone, is responsible to them.

Job descriptions must be worded carefully to ensure that duties are not so narrowly defined that employees will refuse to carry out certain tasks not in their job description.

Alternatively, you might decide to write a job description based on a deficiency in your service. For example, you find that your shop is very untidy. On assessing the reason why, you find that the current staff do not have time to undertake cleaning tasks. You therefore decide to employ a cleaner.

Once you know the activities or tasks that constitute the job, then you are in a position to write a job description. A job description also identifies the tasks and the time allocated to those tasks and this provides the worker with increased autonomy, reducing the need for constant supervision. A job description provides an opportunity for job enhancement by increasing worker independence and it should be used as a management tool throughout the employment to review performance and evaluate further activities.

Items that should be included in a job description are job title, location, job summary, duties, equipment if any, materials and forms used, supervision, working conditions and hazards (to comply with the Health and Safety Acts).

QUESTION 57: LOCUM PAY

I employ a locum pharmacist on an irregular basis. I have always given him his locum fee gross. My accountant is concerned that this may not be correct and perhaps I should treat him as an employee and process him through PAYE. If I do this he is unlikely to stay with me. What can I do?

ANSWER

This has always been an unclear area but in a recent ruling involving Boots The Chemists the Inland Revenue stated that it is alright to pay a locum gross. This requires the locum to be registered with the Inland Revenue as self-employed and therefore liable to pay his/her own Income Tax and National Insurance.

QUESTION 58: WORK CLOTHING

I read in the newspaper that work clothing is not allowable against expenses. Does this include my staff uniforms and my white coat?

ANSWER

There has been a ruling on a case brought to the High Court by a lady barrister who wished to claim against tax for the clothes she wore in court. The ruling made it clear that clothing worn outside the work place could not be claimed against tax.

It is unlikely that you will wear your white coat, or your staff their uniforms, outside work, therefore a tax inspector would have to allow them as legitimate expenses.

QUESTION 59: KEEPING ACCOUNTS

I have just taken over a business and enjoy dealing with customers but I never seem to have time to get my accounts into order. What should I do and is that not my accountant's job anyway?

ANSWER

You appear to have a problem managing your time and you must take steps to get control of it. Take a few minutes to consider what you do during the day. These are some suggestions on how you might better manage your time.

- do the right things
- do things 95% right first time
- delegate
- ignore the telephone
- restrict access to yourself
- create a time saving culture
- prioritize work
- plan work
- set up an efficient retrieval system.

The efficiency and profitability of any business will depend on the quality of its day-to-day management. To be an effective manager you will need to have readily accessible financial information. Additionally, as pharmacy owner, you are responsible by law for ensuring that certain records are maintained. It is vital to establish a reliable book-keeping method from day one, to record daily cash handling and all the financial activities of the business. A number of accounting books are available and are reasonably priced, e.g. Simplex D (George Vyner Ltd). With the availability of computers in pharmacies it is also possible to purchase an inexpensive business computer program such as Sage or Observe (available from the National Pharmaceutical Association). Depending on the complexity of the book or computer program it may also be possible to deal with VAT, wages and accounts in a form acceptable to the Inland Revenue.

At the end of the financial year your accountant will need the books to make up your accounts. If your accounts are well kept this will reduce the amount of time that he works on the books and the costs you pay.

QUESTION 60: RECONCILING ACCOUNTS

I really hate keeping my accounts. How often should I reconcile my accounts?

ANSWER

Love it or hate it accounts are the measure of how successful your business is. Failure to address your accounts on a regular basis means that you will be unaware of what is going on; for example if discrepancies are occurring, or if you are approaching a cash-flow crisis that requires you to take remedial action. Failure to take this action could be very expensive and may show you to be an inefficient manager to your bank.

Your till should be cashed up daily and you should bank your takings at least weekly, or more frequently if you are dealing with large amounts of cash. When banking your takings you should ensure that the money you are lodging, plus the cash that you paid out for wages and services and what you are keeping as a float, balances. This can easily be done in your accounts book. If it does not balance something is wrong and it allows you to remedy the problem there and then.

You should ensure that your bank issues you with a statement of account at least monthly and you should take the time to check that your accounts book is up-to-date ensuring that all direct debits and standing orders are included in your accounts. This will allow you, each month, to have a clear picture of what business is like and will show you how much cash you have in the bank.

When a business is improving, for example, you can become complacent in thinking that since the cash receipts have improved then all must be well with the bank account. However, if this up-turn in business requires more stock to be purchased you could be heading for a cash-flow problem. This can only be predicted if your accounts are constantly kept up-to-date.

QUESTION 61: MONTHLY PRESCRIPTION SUMMARY SHEET

What type of information should I be attempting to establish from my Health Authority (CSA in Northern Ireland amd Health Board in Scotland) monthly statement on my prescription payments?

ANSWER

You will be familiar with the main statistics given on your prescription payment summary report. The following can also be useful statistics to calculate.

- *Average cost of a prescription* is simply the net ingredient cost divided by the number of prescriptions. The lower this value is the more fees you are receiving for money invested in medicines. There is more profit from dispensing where the value is less than £8.70 – the average cost of a medicine.
- *Percentage profit on return* gives you some idea of the profit you are making from NHS dispensing. You add up the amount for fees and professional allowance (say £3800) and divide it by the total of the account (excluding oxygen) (say £22 000). The profit on return is therefore 17.27% for the core dispensing business.

QUESTION 62: NHS PAYMENTS

Why does my NHS payment fluctuate from month to month when I dispense a similar number of prescriptions each month?

ANSWER

The NHS payment each month is not the payment in respect of one month's prescriptions. For England and Wales it comprises an estimated 80% advance for the prescriptions sent to the PPA (or Welsh Pricing Bureau) approximately one month earlier, plus the balance of the value of the prescriptions submitted two months earlier.

As the value of the advance payment is based on the average value of the prescriptions for the previous month any fluctuations in ingredient cost (both up and down) have a double effect on the total payment.

Average ingredient cost per prescription while usually moving in a steady upward trend can have seasonal variations, e.g. it is usually highest in August (because of holidays) and March (because of the end of the financial year).

QUESTION 63: CALCULATING ADVANCE PAYMENTS

How can I check my advance payment calculation?

ANSWER

For England and Wales the advance payment is calculated as follows:

Advance payment for February prescriptions $= (a \times b \times i \times 80\%) - c$

Where
a = contractor's declared number of items for February
b = contractor's average cost per item for January prescriptions
c = inflation factor of 1.01%
i = contractor's declared number of paid items × £5.25.

QUESTION 64: OUT-OF-POCKET EXPENSES

Last Sunday I was on rota and received a prescription for a cylinder of oxygen. I am not an oxygen contractor but since the patient's husband was distressed and the pharmacist who normally supplied this patient was not available I drove to the local British Oxygen Corporation (BOC) depot and got a bottle of oxygen from them in the name of my colleague. Will I be paid if I submit the prescription to the Health Authority?

ANSWER

The short answer is that you will not get paid since you are not in contract with your Health Authority to provide an oxygen service. This would indeed be hard-hearted and the Health Authority would normally treat oxygen as a drug and pay you accordingly. You would also have the right to claim out-of-pocket expenses for your trip to BOC. You should detail these in a letter to your local pharmacy practice committee. You will be paid out-of-pocket expenses for any justifiable expense you incur in providing patients with their medicines.

QUESTION 65: PARTNERSHIPS

I have just got to the end of my first year of trading and have submitted my accounts to my accountant. He has suggested that I make my wife a partner in the business. Can I do that?

ANSWER

If your wife is a pharmacist then there is no reason why you should not make her a partner and there can be a reduction in the amount of Income Tax you will jointly pay, as less will be paid at 40%. Pharmacies can only be owned and operated by a pharmacist, a partnership where all the partners are pharmacists and/or a body corporate.

If your wife is not a pharmacist then you could not legally trade as a partnership under the pharmacy legislation and since the accounts you submit must refer to the legal trading organization this would not be possible.

Personal finance

QUESTION 66: TAX FOR SELF-EMPLOYED

I have owned my own pharmacy for ten months. I have been very careful to keep my drawings from the business as low as possible. Will I only be taxed on the money I take out of the business for my personal use?

ANSWER

The tax due for the business is determined by the net profits earned, adjusted for taxation purposes. There are certain disallowed items such as entertaining and depreciation is added back for tax purposes and set against capital allowances on fixtures and fittings. If you let the profit sit in the business you will still pay tax on it. For example, if you make £50 000 net profit per year for four years and only spend £10 000 per year you are taxed on £50 000 per year. If in the fifth year you only have a net profit of £10 000 but decided to spend £60 000 (this money is lying in the business) you are only taxed on £10 000.

There are two types of tax for businesses – Income Tax which you pay on your income and Capital Gains Tax which is due on the capital generated in the business, such as fixtures and fittings and the property if you are lucky enough to own it.

QUESTION 67: PENSION PLANS FOR WIVES

I have had a pension plan running for some years now and I wish to take a plan out for my wife. Can I do this within my business and get tax relief on the payments?

ANSWER

Yes. Where your wife is employed by the business, even on a part-time basis and no tax or NIC is payable you can opt to start a pension plan for her within the business. The company selling the plan will process the application to the Inland Revenue and you must provide your accountant with a PPCC form stating the nature of the policy and that it qualifies for tax exemption.

QUESTION 68: SELLING A BUSINESS

I am a 58-year-old pharmacist and I wish to retire. I have some savings and I own my own house and business. I estimate that I will make £100000 from the sale of the building and £100000 from the sale of the business. I bought the building in 1975 for £20000 and I paid £6000 for the fixtures and fittings and goodwill. What are the tax implications of selling my business at this time?

ANSWER

Your gains have been good over the years with £80000 on the building and £94000 on the business – so your total gains are £174000.

Since you are over the age of 55 and have owned the business and building for over ten years you can sell your assets and will not be subject to Capital Gains Tax up to £250000. You will not have to pay Capital Gains Tax. If you have made more from the sale of your business you would only be required to pay 50% of Capital Gains Tax on the next £750000 above £250000, i.e. up to £1 million. If you have a long-standing pension plan you will find that your fund – due to its size now at the age of 58 – will increase significantly over the new few years up to the age of 65. Therefore it would be most prudent to retire on the tax-free benefits of the sale of your business and not cash in your pension fund until you are 65.

QUESTION 69: TRANSFER OF CAPITAL GAINS TO WIFE

I have sold my business and now wish to transfer some of the money to my wife. Will she be eligible for tax?

ANSWER

No. Transfer of capital gains between husband and wife, when they are living together, is exempt from Capital Gains Tax. It is probably a good idea to do this as your wife and yourself can both gift an amount of £150 000 to your children. This can help to avoid Inheritance Tax.

QUESTION 70: CHILD MINDING

I have taken a few years off to have my children and I would now like to return to work. I have been offered a pharmacy manageress' position and this will require me to employ a baby minder/housekeeper. Can I obtain tax relief on what I pay my child-minder?

ANSWER

No. This is not regarded as a business expense in the same way as travelling to work is not regarded as a legitimate business expense. Where child minding facilities, such as crèche facilities, are provided to employees by employers, the employer can get some relief but they would not apply in your case.

QUESTION 71: CLAIMING FOR HOME EXPENSES

I own four pharmacies and use a converted bedroom in my house as an office. I often work in this office and keep my invoices etc. there. Is this something that I should be claiming tax relief for?

ANSWER

Yes it is. If this is a genuine office a claim for part of the running costs would be proper. To calculate the amount of expenses you could claim you would have to establish the total cost of running your home which would include lighting, heating, cleaning, insurance etc. You would not be allowed to include the cost of providing an extension to the property.

A fraction would be applied to this total cost of running your home which would take into account the size of the office and the percentage of your time that you spend there. Separate arrangements may need to be made for telephone calls made on behalf of the business and this would include the cost of telephone line rental.

In many cases the pharmacy may have living accommodation attached in which the pharmacist lives or which is given to a pharmacy manager. A clear distinction must be made between what expenses are involved for living accommodation and what is used for running the business. If the shop is on the same heating system for example, or if they share a common telephone line, these issues will need to be taken into account.

QUESTION 72: CONFERENCE EXPENSES

I own and run a pharmacy in the North of England. I attended a Numark Conference in Barcelona this year and my wife, a non-pharmacist, came along. Can I claim tax relief for both my wife and myself for attending this conference?

ANSWER

This is a most unclear situation. There is clearly justification for you as a practising pharmacist to attend this conference but whether a tax inspector is willing to accept the expenses incurred in taking your wife is a different matter. The measure they usually apply is whether the expense is 'wholly, exclusively and necessarily' a part of the business. It could be difficult in fact for you to show that attendance at the conference was really necessary for the running of your business. Different tax inspectors may treat the same claim differently.

Taking your wife's attendance, you would need to show that her presence was necessary. For example, does she decide on some aspects of purchasing for the pharmacy which was dealt with at the conference. If your wife cannot be shown to be associated with the conference then the tax inspector is likely to view the conference as a holiday and disallow relief.

QUESTION 73: PROFESSIONAL EXPENSES/EXAMINATION FEES

I am keen to develop my professional role and have joined the College of Pharmacy Practice. There is a fee for membership of the college and an examination fee for sitting my examinations in the summer. Can I claim both of these items as tax relief?

ANSWER

You may be able to claim the cost of membership of a professional body relating to your profession as a tax deductible expense. You would not however be allowed to claim for examination fees. The Inland Revenue views examination fees as not strictly expenses for running your pharmacy – they are not wholly, exclusively or necessarily part of running the business. They view running your practice and getting an additional professional qualification as different matters. Your fees for membership of the Royal Pharmaceutical Society would be necessary as you could not open the pharmacy door without a registered pharmacist being present. This would also allow you to claim RPharmS registration fees for any full-time pharmacist you employ if you pay their fees.

QUESTION 74: INHERITANCE TAX

I have just retired and have sold my business. My estate is now worth in excess of £500 000. I am suffering from angina and fear that, if I die in the next few years, my estate will be subject to considerable Capital Gains Tax. How might I minimize the charge to Inheritance Tax (IHT)?

ANSWER

The threshold over which IHT is levied is £200 000 for the year 1995–6 and above this limit tax will be charged at 40%. However, if you die within seven years there will be a tax liability. This will depend on when you die. For example, if you die within three years of gifting money your estate or the recipient will pay 100% of full death charge, whereas if you die over six years from the date on which you gifted money your estate or the recipient will only pay tax at 20% of full death charge.

If you divide your estate with your wife then this allows either of you to give your children up to £200 000. If one of you dies in the next few years this allows the other to transfer this amount to your children tax-free. This would then leave the balance to the spouse free of IHT under the surviving spouse exemption.

You can also elect to give annual lifetime transfers of up to £3000 each per year, i.e. you could give away £6000 between you and your wife. If you have not made gifts in the previous year you can carry this forward and give away an additional £6000 for a total of £12 000 in all. It is also possible to give away £250 each in separate gifts over and above that limit. You can also make additional gifts in consideration of marriage to the bride and/or groom – up to £5000 by a parent, £2500 by a grandparent or £1000 by any other person.

QUESTION 75: INHERITANCE TAX MANAGEMENT

My wife has just died and I retired three years ago. In my will I left all my estate to my wife. I have four grown-up children. How should I make provision for them?

ANSWER

You could make use of the gifts to remove some of your estate. However, when you die your estate may be chargeable for the full amount of IHT. You would be well-advised to obtain estate-planning advice in order to minimize IHT at some time in the future. First you should contact your accountant who will be in a position to recommend someone qualified to give independent financial advice.

QUESTION 76: MEDICAL INSURANCE POLICIES

I am a 38-year-old pharmacist and I am currently building up my business. I bought my second pharmacy this year. I am a member of the Pharmacy Mutual Insurance scheme. I am not sure about all the advantages of this scheme but I know that it will provide me with the cost of a locum if I am unable to work due to illness. The person who has sold me a pension plan is now trying to interest me in a policy that will provide me with sickness cover. It is a package that will pay me a lump sum if I find that I am suffering from one of a number of chronic conditions such as heart disease. I am also a member of BUPA. I am confused about the advantage of taking out this extra cover. Will it be of advantage to me and who can advise?

ANSWER

The law is now very strict in respect of who can give financial advice. You should ensure that the advice you get is independent. From what you say it does not seem that the person attempting to interest you in this sickness package is independent and is probably linked to one of the major insurance groups.

You are wise to have as many 'defenders' as you can if you are developing your business as illness could greatly restrict your performance and although you and your partner are in the best of health, sickness can strike at any time.

The Pharmacy Mutual is a dedicated scheme for pharmacists and you should have the maximum number of shares in this scheme which will allow you to get through most episodes of ill-health and keep your business running as smoothly as possible. The annual premium that you pay to the scheme is not allowed against tax and any payments made from the scheme must also be taxed. On retirement, presuming that you continue to pay into the scheme, you will receive a tax-free lump sum irrespective of the amount of sickness payments you have claimed.

The premiums for the scheme that is being offered to you at this time will not be exempt from tax.

If you employ your wife in the pharmacy you could claim her portion of any BUPA fee in the same way as you claim her pension contributions. So long as your wife is not paid more than £8500 per year the cost to you to provide these benefits will not be taxed upon her.

You must decide if you feel that the extra security you are being offered would be of benefit. Contact an independent financial adviser.

QUESTION 77: TAX AND MARITAL SEPARATION

I am a pharmacy manager and have recently got divorced after two years of being legally separated. It has been a difficult time and I have not considered all the implications. My ex-wife and I had no children. I appear to still be receiving a married man's allowance. How should I get my tax code changed?

ANSWER

From the time that you no longer live with, or wholly maintain, your wife you cannot claim a married man's allowance. Therefore from the time that you were legally separated your tax code should have been changed. Your employer can organize this to be done for you. You will need to repay the married man's relief that you received from the time that you were legally separated and this might be done by changing your tax code so that HM Inspector of Taxes (HMIT) can recoup the Income Tax that you owe them.

QUESTION 78: TAXATION ON PENSIONS

I shall be retiring in two years time and have a pension plan which I have been paying into for most of my working life. I intend to take part of my pension as a lump sum (25%) and the rest of the fund I will take annually to live on. What tax will I pay?

ANSWER

Normally your lump sum will be free of tax but it may not relate to 25% of your pension fund. If you invest the money you will be taxed on the money that you make from these investments. The monthly pension payments you receive will be subject to tax in the same way as your income was before you took retirement.

If you continue to work as a locum pharmacist this will be regarded as income and will attract tax. You could only claim justifiable expenses against the money that you earn as a locum and not against the money paid as your pension. For example, if you wished to remain a member of the Royal Pharmaceutical Society you would be able to claim your registration fee against your income but not against your pension.

QUESTION 79: TAX-FREE INVESTMENTS

On my retirement I received a considerable lump sum. I now would like to invest this. Are there any areas in which I can invest this money so that the interest avoids tax at the higher rate?

ANSWER

You might consider an investment that produces capital growth or one that generates a return that is exempt from Income Tax.

National Savings Certificates offer a reasonable return up to a gross equivalent of about 10% that is non-taxable. There are also index-linked National Savings Scheme Certificates that you might consider. The minimum purchase is £25 and the maximum holding is £5000 but this applies to each issue and you can hold a similar amount in other issues.

The index-linked issue can be bought in units of £25 up to a maximum of £10000. The return on these issues, which is totally tax-free, is calculated by the rise in inflation as measured by the retail price index. To this factor is added a further percentage for all certificates that are held to a maturity of five years. For someone who is a 40% tax-payer and estimating a 10% gain tax-free this is equivalent to a gross yield of 16.7%.

Premium Savings Bonds are still available up to a maximum saving of £10000. Any prize that might be won is entirely free of tax and your money is safe.

Personal Equity Plans (PEPs) were introduced some years ago to encourage tax-payers to invest in company shares. The limit for investment for any one year is £6000 and although this is not available for actual tax relief, the income you receive from it and any consequential capital gains that might arise, are entirely free of all taxes. If you die in ownership of a PEP, however, your estate will be required to pay IHT on any gains.

You might consider transferring monies to your wife if she is not a tax-payer and to your children. Because they are not tax-payers they can gain interest free of tax up to a certain amount.

QUESTION 80: WAGES FOR WIFE

My wife works in the home and I put her through the books as a part-time member of staff and put a salary in for her. Is this OK?

ANSWER

HMIT would first wish to know what work your wife did for the business to justify this wage. There is no question that she works hard within the home but if she takes no part in the business then the wage would not be justified. Where your wife is involved in the business, for example doing the accounts, there would need to be some proof that the wage is given over to her rather than simply being a paper transaction.

QUESTION 81: INCOME TAX – SELF-EMPLOYED

I have been in business for 18 months and I have just received my first tax bill which has come as quite a shock. The payment will be due within 30 days of the date of issue yet I expected it to be due in January which is six months away. Due to the considerable investment I have made I find that I may not be able to pay this bill. What are my options?

ANSWER

Your accountant will be able to guide you on whether the tax bill is accurate. If it is your first assessment then it will be due within 30 days. The next assessments will be due in January and July and if the amount is correct you are going to have to pay the bill. HMIT is not going to wait for their money forever and you will be charged interest for late payments. This interest is currently around 8% which is slightly less than the interest you would pay to the bank. The interest is not allowable against tax as it is not a business expense. It is important that you attempt to pay the tax bill when you can.

QUESTION 82: MATERNITY BENEFIT – SELF-EMPLOYED

For ten years, up until last year, I was an employee pharmacist working full-time for a multiple pharmacy group. This year I bought a pharmacy which I now run. Recently I got married and I now find I am expecting a baby. I have been told that as a self-employed person I cannot receive statutory maternity pay (SMP). Is this correct?

ANSWER

Yes. SMP only applies to employees who pay Class 1 National Insurance Contributions (NICs). You no longer pay this. You will, however, be able to claim a maternity allowance due to the fact that you have paid Class 1 NICs in the last two years. You should contact your local social security office for more information on this.

QUESTION 83: NATIONAL INSURANCE CONTRIBUTIONS (NICS)

I have recently become self-employed and I understand that I must now pay my own NICs but that it is different from the NICs I paid as an employee. Can you explain?

ANSWER

As a self-employed person you will be liable to pay two classes of National Insurance Contributions: (a) the flat rate Class 2 contribution; and (b) the earnings-related Class 4 contribution.

Class 2 contribution is paid either by direct debit from your bank account or quarterly by cheque. This payment is not allowed against tax and is currently £5.85 per week. If you think you are not paying this you should check with your local DSS office quoting your National Insurance number. There is a lower limit for payment of £3310 per year. If you were an employee pharmacist on PAYE and you did some locum work you could get locum pay up to £3310 per year before you were required to pay Class 2 NIC, as well as Class 1 which is taken from your main salary.

Class 4 contributions are paid with your normal half-yearly Income Tax demand. The rate is 7.3% as for 1995-6 on the band of income between £6640 and £22 880 per annum, giving a maximum contribution of £1185.52. If you earn taxable income in excess of £22 880 per annum you will therefore pay this amount.

Class 4 national insurance is 50% tax deductible.

QUESTION 84: LOCUM FEES – PAYE PHARMACISTS

I manage a pharmacy for a multiple chain and over the last few months I have been doing the odd locum duty for colleagues. For this work I get paid £100 gross. I know I must pay tax on this money but how exactly do I do it?

ANSWER

Each year you receive tax form 11 from HMIT that must be completed. On this form there is a section in which you must include any payments you received in addition to your normal salary. If you do not receive this form you must request it from your local tax office.

From time to time the Inland Revenue when checking a pharmacy's accounts will note down the names of those pharmacists who have been paid locum fees. They will then cross-reference this to establish whether you made the declaration on your form. If you have failed to declare additional sources of income you are liable for a fine. Under the new self-assessment scheme for taxation currently being introduced the responsibility for declaration lies with the recipient of the money.

QUESTION 85: COMPANY CARS

I am the manager of a pharmacy and have been looking for a pay rise. My boss has suggested that he will provide me with a car that is probably worth about £2000 a year to me. Is it?

ANSWER

In real terms it is. What you will be getting is a company car and this will be declared in your annual tax returns. Your employer will state on form P11D – the expense return form – the list price of the car and the mileage you do for the business. The Inland Revenue will estimate the value of the car and your code will be changed which effectively means that you will pay additional tax. Don't be put off, a company car should be less expensive than if you had to buy the car yourself. There are three levels of legitimate company car usage – low, medium and high. For a pharmacist it would be difficult to prove that your company car was used a lot for company business. It is likely that you will be eligible for the least number of miles up to 2500 per year. If you are placed in a higher bracket you probably will be asked by HMIT to justify this.

QUESTION 86: PARTNERSHIPS

For tax purposes I made my wife a partner in my business although she had nothing to do with it. We have recently had a legal separation and she is claiming a full 50% share of the business. Is there any way I can minimize the percentage of the business she owns?

ANSWER

If your wife was a partner in the business and she is not a pharmacist you may have been trading illegally. For the purpose of taxation HMIT considers a partnership to be a trade or profession carried out jointly by two or more individuals for the purpose of profit. It is a matter of fact and is not dependent on any written agreement. If you say your wife was not playing any part in the business then in fact she cannot be a partner. The difficulty you have is that technically you have been falsifying your accounts over the years by claiming a partnership existed when in fact it did not.

If the business accounts that have been accepted by the Inland Revenue shows your wife to be a 50% partner in the business it is going to be very difficult for you to prove otherwise. She will have a 50% claim to the assets (possessions) of the business.

$$\text{Total assets} = \frac{\text{Total liabilities}}{(\text{Owner's equity} + \text{Creditors owing})}$$

QUESTION 87: TAX RELIEF ON WIFE'S CAR

I am buying a car for my wife. What tax might I save against my business expenses?

ANSWER

The short answer is none. I presume that you have your own car and that certain business expenses are set against it which will give tax relief. In the case where your wife is not a partner in the business the Inland Revenue would view your wife's car as having no value to the business.

Accounts are prepared to reflect business activities solely and not the private activities of the proprietor or the shareholders. As a general concept the Inland Revenue will always consider if something is wholly, exclusively and necessarily used for the business when considering an expense for tax reasons.

INDEX

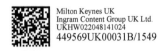

Milton Keynes UK
Ingram Content Group UK Ltd.
UKHW022048141024
449569UK00031B/1549